The "No Diet" Diet

How to get the body you want while still eating whatever you want

BY: CARLO MACAPINLAC

Disclaimer

No part of this publication may be reproduced or transmitted in any form by any means without permission in writing from the author and publisher.

This book is meant for educational purposes only. You are responsible for determining your own nutritional, medical, and psychological needs. Please consult with your doctor before making any changes to your diet or beginning any exercise program.

The author is not a licensed medical care provider and represents that he has no expertise in diagnosing, examining, or treating medical conditions of any kind or in determining the effect of any specific exercise on a medical condition. The information in this book is based on my own personal experience and my interpretation of available data.

You should understand that, when participating in any exercise or exercise program, there is the possibility of physical injury.

If you engage in the exercise or exercise program in this book, you agree that you do so at your own risk, are voluntarily participating in these activities, assume all risk of injury to yourself, and agree to release and discharge the author and publisher from any and all claims or causes of action, known or unknown, arising out of the author and publisher's negligence.

Dedication

This book is dedicated to my brother, Myke. Thank you for dragging my butt, kicking and screaming, to the local YMCA many years ago. Little did I know that it would open the door to a completely different life.

I also want to dedicate this book to my family. Mom, Dad, and Jean—thanks for always being my biggest fans.

To all my friends, coaches, and training partners—I love you all. Thank you for inspiring me to be 1% better every day.

Table of Contents

"Actually, I just woke up one day and decided I didn't want to feel like that anymore. Or ever again. So I changed. Just like that." – Unknown

Why I Created This Book and How to Use It

It's lunchtime again at the office.

I make my way to the cafeteria and greet the lunch lady with a smile. She sees me every day. "The usual?" she says. It's taco Tuesday after all. Three chicken tacos, a side of fries, and a can of diet coke. My typical lunch on Tuesdays. After inhaling my meal, I waddle my way to the vending machine and grab a Snickers bar for dessert.

To be quite frank, that was the most exciting part of my day back then.

I showed up to a job I hated every day, drove a car I could barely afford, lived in a cramped apartment, binge-watched TV until some ungodly hour, and wasted away my weekends drinking my face off. Worst of all, I hated how my body looked.

Food was my biggest vice. I turned to food to make myself feel better if I was having a bad day. Why? It's easy and it's delicious.

I would then see my naked body the next day in the shower and I would hate myself even more. Another bad day. But hey, at least it's wing Wednesday at the office cafeteria. I think they also have a new dessert. That should do the trick.

This vicious cycle went on for years and I started to develop what kids these days call a "dad bod."

I was in my early twenties. This is supposed to be the peak years of my physical health, and I was anything but healthy.

I would find some motivation every once in a while, usually at the beginning of the year, to go on a diet, but to no avail. It was hard. I felt deprived. I just enjoyed food way too much so I felt like a failure every single time I slipped out of the diet.

Sound familiar?

I see this everywhere.

People not feeling good about themselves. They want to make a change but they just don't know where to start.

You see people try every diet under the sun and fail miserably. They're back to square one every single time and they're left wondering what went wrong.

After years of trial and error through blood, sweat, and tears, I finally figured it out. I developed a system for getting the body I've always wanted without giving up my favorite food.

Needless to say, my life changed drastically. I finally liked how my body looked. I walked around feeling two inches taller because I had more confidence in myself. People at work started treating me better. I didn't feel like the "invisible man" to women anymore—I actually started getting dates. I became a better weekend warrior because I was in better shape.

It was if I was a new man. What people don't realize is that health isn't about the weight you lose but about the life you gain.

Even after helping other people get similar and even better results with my system, I still had a lot of self-limiting beliefs about why I should write a book on dieting. But then I realized I'm not really on a diet. I'm still able to enjoy the food I love. That's how the "No Diet" Diet was born.

This is my way of giving back to the world. It's my way of answering all the questions I had when I was just starting out and helping people like my old self take that first step to getting healthy and finally figuring out this endless cycle of dieting and failing once and for all.

This is something I wish I had back then. Life is hard enough as it is, and I want to give people a fighting chance. If you pick up just one or two things from this book that make your life 1% better, then I've done my job as an author.

Listen, there's no perfect time to do something. Stop waiting until you feel like you're ready to change.

Just remember that you're one decision away from a completely different life.

Oversimplistic? Probably.

But I think there's a lot of truth to that statement. Sometimes it all starts with simply making a decision to change. If you're reading this book right now, then you've already taken that all-important step.

But in order for all of this to work, you have to take action. If you just read through this book but don't take action, it's kind of like going to the gym and having someone explain to you what running on a treadmill is like or how to exercise without actually doing it. Reading about it and feeling good about yourself simply isn't enough. Nobody has ever achieved their goals just by reading about it.

Long story short, you need to put all the information you learn from this book to good use. There's gonna be action steps at the end of some chapters, and it's all about following through with it.

At the end of the day, your life will come down to your decisions, and if you change your decisions, you will change everything.

Are you ready? Let's go.

Introduction

43,261,543.

That's not just a random number. I made roughly that many mistakes when I was just starting out this whole fitness thing.

I spent a lot of time searching the far depths of the Internet and looking for that elusive magic pill to finally getting a flat stomach.

I'll give you a hint: it doesn't exist.

Who could blame us? We're all busy people. We all have things to do, whether it's your job, school (or both), trying to maintain your social life, taking care of your dog, or watching Netflix. The list goes on and on.

Life gets in the way sometimes. Scratch that: when it comes to getting fit, it gets in the way most of the time.

We make as many as 200 decisions when it comes to food alone every day.

Then you're fed with things like "breakfast is the most important meal of the day," "don't forget to drink a glass of orange juice," "eat a small meal every three hours," "you should go low fat," or "you should go vegan." It's easy for things to get overwhelming.

There's so many voices and "experts" out there selling you the next best thing about weight loss, you don't really know who to trust.

Paralysis by analysis kicks in, so you end up doing nothing.

No wonder most people don't make it past January when it comes to keeping their fitness New Year's resolution.

Hey, you can always try next year, right?

The thing is, anybody can work out for an hour every day. That alone can be quite an achievement. It's what you do with the other 23 hours that greatly determines your results.

Think about it.

That hour-long workout is only 4% of your day. What are you doing with the other 96%? Yet most people only focus on the exercise part and just hit cruise control for the rest of the day.

The problem is, you can't outrun a bad diet.

We live in a world of instant gratification, so we turn to weight loss pills, crash diets, and juice cleanses for fast results. I even saw an ad the other day about "freezing" your fat away. Good luck with that.

The fact is, there is simply no overnight fix when it comes to losing fat.

If it were easy, everybody would look like they just came off the set of *Baywatch*.

Sadly, it's not.

If you picked up this book and hoped to find the magic elixir to weight loss, then you should probably stop reading and ask for a refund now.

What I am about to show you in this book are the key principles I've learned during the last six years that've helped me get to where I am today. They're the same principles I teach my students at Newbie Fitness Academy.

I've spent that last few years trying to figure out what works and what doesn't. I sorted out through all the BS in the world of fitness and I've found that there are really only four key parts you need to focus on:

1. Mindset
2. Sleep
3. Nutrition
4. Exercise

For this system to work, you need to have all four parts working in unison. Miss out on one and the sum isn't as effective.

This book isn't about reinventing the wheel of fitness.

You've probably already heard some of the things I'm going to talk about. Some of the material might be new to you as well.

But there are two keys things to all of this:

1. It's all about having an open mind for trying new things and getting over old beliefs and stories that are backed up by nothing but cooler talk and bro-science.

2. It's one thing to read about all the things I'm about to teach you. It's another thing to take action. And it's all about taking action. I could reveal to you the secret to eternal life, but if you don't take action, then it's worth nothing.

At the end of the day, it's all about having a sustainable system that you can rely on for the rest of your life and not having to worry about dieting.

Follow through with the core principles of this book and you're going to be further ahead than 99% of the population hoping and praying that their dream body will come knocking on their door one day.

Part 1: Mindset

"Anything worth doing is worth doing well." – Hunter S. Thompson

Chapter 1: The Most Important Question You Need to Ask Yourself

Often neglected but crucial nonetheless.

People often miss the boat on this.

Let's start with one of my favorite quotes by Victor Frankl. He says, "He who has a why to live for can bear almost any how."

Translation: if you have an unbelievable desire to accomplish something, you will move mountains to achieve it, no matter what the circumstances are.

A huge part of your success is going to depend on knowing why you want to lose weight to begin with.

Why are you here? Why do you want to change?

Knowing your *why* will then help you create a solid foundation to develop a strong mindset, which is probably going to be the most important tool in your journey.

You could have the best diet, the best meal plan, or the best workouts laid out for you, but if your mind isn't in the right space, you're simply not gonna get the results you're looking for.

The moment you encounter that first obstacle—and there will be many—you're always going to find the path of least resistance, and that usually means giving up on your goals and going back to your old habits.

Why? Because it's easy. It's comfortable. You're used to it.

I believe that this is one of the biggest reasons why people fail when they're trying to lose weight.

They just don't have a strong enough *why*.

When You're Down, the Only Way Is Up

Finding my *why* came to me at a pretty low point in my life.

It came at a time when I just got laid off from my engineering job, my long-term relationship just ended, and I was in the worst shape of my life. Looking back now, maybe that's why she dumped me.

All of a sudden, I was back to being single, I was lonely, I was out of a job, and my health, fitness, and general sense of well-being were in a terrible place. I didn't feel good about myself, to say the least.

Because of this, my self-esteem suffered, my social circle dwindled, and my dating life was obviously nonexistent.

I started to feel needy and desperate. I felt like I wasn't good enough. I didn't feel like doing anything. I felt lost. The thought of leaving the house, let alone my room at times, seemed like an impossible task.

I turned to food for comfort, and it caused me to gain even more weight. I hated my body every time I looked at myself in the mirror. I would purposely avoid going to public places where I had to take my shirt off in front of other people because I didn't want them to see me shirtless.

I turned down every invitation I got when it came to anything that involved physical exertion; I was afraid I was gonna make a fool of myself in front of everyone because I wasn't fit.

I bought clothes that were one size too big just so I could hide my man boobs.

Sound familiar?

Life sucked, to say the least.

Then, one day, the pain of remaining the same finally became greater than the pain of making a change in my life. I just got to a point where I was just sick and tired of being sick and tired. That became my *why*.

So I changed. But it's not always as simple as that for a lot of people.

It's Your Turn

Now, you need to ask yourself why you're doing this. Really dig deep on this one.

Let your *why* fuel your fire.

It could be about finally having the confidence to ask out the girl or guy you've always liked.

It could be about wanting to become a better weekend warrior.

It could be about being fit enough to play catch with your kid without throwing out your back.

It could be about having the courage to finally ask for that promotion you think you deserve or maybe finally having the guts to quit your job and switch careers.

It could be as simple as finally being able to fit in the clothes you want to wear and not have to buy baggy clothes to hide your body.

It could be about finally liking the person you see in the mirror.

Or maybe you're just like me and you're just sick and tired of feeling crappy about yourself.

Life sucks and you're finally ready to make a change. I mean, when you're at a very low point in your life like I was a few years ago, the only way to go is up.

Once you find out your *why*, only then will you understand what matters and what doesn't. Only then can you say no when everyone else says yes.

ACTION STEPS

Find out your *why*.

Chapter 2: Why Motivation Is Garbage and What to Do Instead

Motivation is everything.

At least, that's what everyone says.

You probably have all these great ideas in your head about finally making a change and losing weight, but if you feel like you need motivation to do it, then you're doing it wrong.

By watching enough motivational videos, we've bought into this lie that you've gotta feel ready in order to change.

We bought into this complete falsehood that at some point you're gonna have the courage to change. At some point, you're gonna have the confidence to finally dive in.

At some point, you're gonna feel "ready" to do it.

You have these incredible ideas, and what you think you need is motivation to finally get started.

Unfortunately, nothing could be further from the truth.

A quick search on Google and you get 24 million hits on the term "New Year's resolution."

That's a lot. But not surprising. But what were all these people doing during the other 364 days of the year?

Why wait so long?

Why wait until January 1?

Did you know that over one-third of resolutions don't make it past the end of the January?

And only 8% of people actually keep their New Year's resolutions. Barely one in ten. I'm not big on gambling, but those aren't very good odds.

Why? Because people rely solely on motivation to power them through. That's great. The problem is, we only have a finite amount of it. Then it runs out.

That's when things start to get interesting.

Think about it. When your motivation juices are running high, it's easy to get things done, right? Getting started is always the easiest part. But what happens when your motivation runs dry after a few days or after a few weeks?

Let's use fitness, for example. You're finally ready to lose weight and get that elusive six pack.

So you look up the "best" diet on the Internet. You start buying healthy food. You start meal prepping. You sign up for a gym membership. Things are going great.

But then, one day, you're just having one of those really bad days. Maybe you had a long day at work. You don't feel like working out. Somebody brought lefto-ver treats to the office. Your dog ate your favorite workout shirt.

All of a sudden, it's not so easy to stick to your plan anymore. You start getting demotivated, and this is the beginning of the end.

This is when people start to fall off the wagon.

The next day, you start going out for lunch instead of eating your grilled chicken and steamed broccoli. You start going to the kitchen office more often because that's where the free donuts are stashed. You start to find every reason to skip the gym.

Next thing you know, you're completely off the wagon and you're back to square one.

This is why you shouldn't rely on sheer motivation alone. Everyone has good days and bad days, and our actions shouldn't always just be dictated by how moti-vated we're feeling that day.

It's what you do on the days when you don't feel like sticking to your plan that matters the most.

Life happens. I get it.

But that's where discipline comes in.

Discipline is knowing the difference between what you want now and what you want the most.

And being disciplined comes from having a strong *why*. Being disciplined repeatedly over time then brings consistency, and consistency brings results.

Let me repeat. Consistency over time is what gets you results.

For example, you didn't sleep well the night before and you're not having a good start to your day. That's a pretty easy excuse to just eat crap and start fresh tomorrow, right? We're emotional eaters, after all. And hey, there's always tomorrow.

But it's what you do today despite how you feel that will eventually bring the results you want.

That's where discipline and consistency come into play.

Change takes time. Getting a six pack is a process, but the most important part is the process. Learn to love the journey. There's always a lesson to be learned in every situation.

It took you months, if not years, to get to where you're at today. So you shouldn't expect to just change completely overnight. There's no shortcut to all this.

Strive to be better every day, not just at the beginning of the year when you make your New Year's resolutions.

Just remember, you don't need any more motivation. What you need is a solid plan and the knowledge to act, regardless of how motivated you are.

Chapter 3: Why You Need to Stop Looking at Other People's Progress Pictures

We've all seen it.

Everybody including their dog is on social media these days and showing off their "progress" pictures with some motivational quote that reads somewhere along the lines of "What's your excuse?"

We're constantly bombarded with it.

The thing is, very few people actually look like that when they're just walking around in their everyday lives.

Want some proof? Here's my three-second "transformation":

Go to:

>>>   www.newbiefitnessacademy.com/threesecond-transformation

Both pictures were taken literally seconds apart. On the left is me fully relaxed. The picture on the right is me inhaling and fully flexing my abs.

Big difference, right?

The lighting, angle, your posture, whether you've eaten that day, and maybe adding an Instagram filter or two can change the way your body looks completely.

Let's be honest. Most people look more like the picture on the left. I look like the picture on the left 90% of the time.

But because the six pack "progress" picture is what gets circulated on social media (go check your Facebook or Instagram right now and you'll find one within seconds), it creates this awful body stereotype that you feel like you have to live up to. Plus, nobody really posts pictures of themselves sitting on the couch and showing their fat rolls. Everyone just wants to show off their "progress."

It makes people feel like they must be doing something wrong if they're not close to looking like the aforementioned "after" picture. It makes people feel like they're not doing enough when they see their friends' hiking or surfing pictures.

Someone might always be posting pictures of the green smoothies they drink or the fancy-looking salad they had for lunch, yet they might spend the rest of their day eating Nutella out of the jar. You just never know.

Social media only puts you in a place of lack, especially when it comes to your progress. It creates more harm than good.

According to research, a typical teenage girl in the United Kingdom spends an average of 12 minutes getting ready for every selfie they take [1].

That's a mind-blowing one hour and 24 minutes every week—just to get ready for that perfect shot! Think about how many selfies some people take throughout the day.

The bottom line is, just don't believe all the hype you see online. Spend less time on social media and more in real life, where everyone's life is far from the picture-perfect Instagram-filtered world that's portrayed on your screen.

I used to be a victim of this "before and after" progress phenomenon. I was addicted to what people thought of my progress on social media. One day, I finally realized how unhealthy this behavior was to my own personal happiness, so I deleted all social media apps on my phone. I just wanted to see what life would be like without the constant pressure of trying to keep up with everyone.

As I write this chapter, I'm now approaching day 50 of zero social media interaction. It's literally one of the best things I've ever done for myself. It made me focus on the moment, and it took away all the pressure of always trying to show my best self on social media. I'm much happier now because I've just been focusing on my own journey. I'm now more connected with myself instead of the collective thoughts of whomever I was connected with through social media. I'm now more present than ever.

I'm not saying that you should delete social media forever. I think it has its place in today's society in terms of making connections with people all over the world.

But I want you to just focus on your own journey. Focus on progress, not perfection. Don't compare your life behind the scenes to someone else's highlight reel.

ACTION STEPS

Try going off the grid for a week. You don't need to deactivate your social media accounts completely, but just delete the apps on your phone. See how much freedom this simple act will give you. It's going to be weird at first. It might even be a struggle for some people. But try it out. You can personally thank me later by sending me an email to info@newbiefitnessacademy.com.

Part 2: Sleep

"Sleep is the best meditation." – Dalai Lama

Chapter 4: You're Screwed if You Don't Get This Part Right

Sleep.

This is your starting point.

This part is so important that, if you don't get it right, you're not gonna see the results you're looking for, even if I give you the best diet advice and the best workouts on the planet.

It's that simple.

If that's news to you, that's a very good indication of why you've had such a hard time losing weight.

Let's pick things up back in 2012. I was already working out around that time, but I wasn't getting the results I wanted. I was getting strong, but the way my body looked didn't really reflect it. I wasn't getting a very good return on my time investment and I couldn't really figure out why.

I bartended at a nightclub to pay the bills, which meant that getting off work at 3:00 a.m. was a regular thing. I went to a lot of parties. I played video games and would often go to bed at some ungodly hour. Sleep back then was basically just an option and not a necessity.

Long story short, I still had no idea what I was doing. I lived off fast food because it's the only thing that's available late at night. Really, I had it at any time because I didn't know any better. It resulted in me gaining weight—a lot of weight.

Sound familiar? I know I'm not alone on that. Most people fall into this trap.

They're under the impression that they can just look up the "best" workout program out there and ignore their sleep and nutrition and expect to get results.

People even look up workouts for specific body parts, thinking they can just spot-treat themselves. The problem is, it doesn't work that way. You can do 100 bicep curls every day, but if you have a lot of fat to lose, you're simply not going to see the results you're looking for. I call this the "hope and pray" method, and you're gonna be hoping and praying for a long time if this is your strategy.

I spent a good chunk of my twenties getting an average of five to six hours of sleep per night and wondered why I always felt like crap, why I couldn't lose weight, why I always had low energy, and why I always seemed to get sick at least once every couple of weeks. Sound familiar?

The thing is, people seem to wear their lack of sleep like a badge of honor, like someone is gonna give them a medal for being tough and pulling off an all-nighter. I mean, that's how you stay productive, right?

No wonder I never considered my lack of sleep to be a problem. I just didn't know any better. I couldn't figure out why I wasn't seeing any results. It turns out, depriving myself of sleep is one of the biggest reasons why.

The Less You Sleep, the More You Weigh

Getting by on five hours of sleep and pulling off an all-nighter isn't a testament to your mental endurance, toughness, and how productive you are. In fact, not getting enough sleep is probably one of the biggest reasons why you're not losing weight. Here's what you need to know about sleep.

According to research, lack of sleep has a direct relation to weight gain (and eventually obesity) and raises your risk of developing heart disease [2].

The term "I'll sleep when I'm dead" will have a whole new meaning to you if you keep ignoring your sleep.

Yet we deprive ourselves of sleep all the time. Here's a few numbers that jump out right away if you don't get enough sleep.

Studies show that over a third of American adults are not getting enough sleep on a regular basis [3].

Why is that important?

When you consider the fact that the obesity rates for men and women in the United States are nearly the same, the relationship between sleep and obesity starts to make a little bit more sense [4].

To put it simply, people who don't get enough sleep at night tend to weigh significantly more than those who get adequate sleep [5].

In fact, lack of sleep is one of the strongest contributors to obesity. In one study, children and adults who were sleep-deprived were 89% and 55% more likely to become obese, respectively [6].

Participants in this study who reported less than five hours of sleep per night had an approximately 40% higher risk of developing obesity than did those who reported seven to eight hours of sleep [7].

A study that recorded the sleep patterns of 9000 people indicated that those who averaged only six hours of sleep per night were 27% more likely to be overweight than those who slept seven to nine hours. The participants who averaged five hours of sleep were 73% more likely to be overweight [8].

Let me repeat that for a second.

Five hours of sleep increases your chances of being overweight by 73 freaking percent!

And if all that wasn't enough, sleep deprivation makes you eat bigger portion sizes, further increasing the likelihood of you gaining weight [9]. It also disrupts the daily fluctuations in appetite hormones and is believed to cause poor appetite regulation [10,11].

You're fighting a losing battle all because you're not getting enough sleep.

Here's where it gets more serious.

A review of 15 studies found that short sleepers are at a far greater risk of heart disease or stroke than those who sleep seven to eight hours per night [12].

In a study of healthy young men, restricting sleep to four hours per night for six nights in a row caused symptoms of pre-diabetes [13].

Yikes.

Sleep is just something that most of us are willing to sacrifice in a heartbeat.

What I do know is that sleep is absolutely necessary to your success. I talk about this first for a reason because it's something that you can fix right away, starting tonight!

Sleep deprivation has so many negative effects on your body that it's impossible to sustainably improve your fitness with nutrition and exercise until you fix your sleep.

If you're wondering why your last attempt at losing weight didn't go according to plan, not getting enough sleep is probably one of the biggest reasons why (and also if you have a crappy diet and don't exercise).

It's just as important as having the right mindset, eating healthy, and working out. You need to have all four working in unison if you want long-term results.

Again, I've never heard anyone complain about actually getting enough sleep at night.

How Much Sleep Do You Actually Need?

Now that we've established how crucial sleep is to your success, we need to find out how much sleep you actually need.

According to the National Sleep Foundation, if you are between the ages of 18 and 65, you need to get anywhere between seven and nine hours of sleep every night.

Cool? Cool.

ACTION STEPS

Captain Obvious here. Get some sleep.

Chapter 5: How to Get Better Sleep

The next logical question then becomes, how do you actually get better sleep?

I could easily tell you to just close your eyes and end this chapter, but you paid good money to get a copy of this book so I'm gonna talk about sleep a little bit more.

There are five key areas that we're gonna focus on. Don't worry about being perfect. Just be good. You can't just change everything overnight.

1. All Black Everything

The more light you remove from your room, the better. Put simply, you need to sleep in a pitch-black room every night.

Your eyes sense any light in the room, even when they're closed. This disrupts the release of melatonin from your body and greatly affects the quality of sleep you get. That's why it's way harder to fall asleep during the day. You know all about this if you do shift work.

The indicator light on the laptop charger next to your bed, that bright display on your alarm clock, the lights on the cable box, your phone and your TV, and the light coming from your bedroom windows all contribute to disrupting your sleep pattern.

You want to eliminate as much light as possible if you want your room to be more conducive to providing you better sleep.

Quick Fix Tips

Get a different alarm clock. You can go old school on this and get an analog alarm clock. Or get rid of your alarm clock completely and just use your phone.

Speaking of phones, set it on *do not disturb* or *sleep* mode when you sleep. The fewer notifications you get, the better. No, you don't need to watch that cat video for the 100th time.

Unplug any gadgets that have indicator lights, or at the very least, try to hide it in plain sight. Again, it's all about making your room as dark as possible.

Invest in blackout curtains or blinds. Notice how you always get the best sleep when you're in a nice hotel room with fancy curtains? That's their secret.

If you're on a budget, you can invest in a sleep mask. Who cares if it looks dorky. No one else will see you (other than your significant other) anyway.

2. Be Consistent

The consistency of your sleep is just as crucial as the amount and quality of sleep you get.

Why?

According to one study [14], graveyard shifts, also known as shift work, are so destructive to your health that it's been categorized by the World Health Organization as a possible carcinogen—yup, the stuff that could potentially cause cancer.

Unfortunately, a lot of people have imposed graveyard shifts on themselves, especially on weekends, when sleep basically becomes just an afterthought.

Your body doesn't act like a rechargeable battery in that you can't just say "I only got five hours of sleep the previous night so I'll just sleep an extra three tonight and call it even." Sometimes it could take you a few days or even the rest of the week to recover from one night of bad sleep.

Here's what to do: avoid sleeping in even on weekends. Try to go to bed at a consistent time every night. I know this might be difficult depending on your circumstances, but at this point you should realize just how crucial this is.

3. What You Put in Your Body Before Bed Matters

We've been conditioned by today's society to eat, drink, and socialize at night. That's fair because most people have jobs during the day. Plus, it's fun!

But what you put in your body, specifically right before you go to bed, has a huge correlation with the type of sleep you're going to get.

This should be pretty obvious, but don't order an almond milk, nonfat, triple shot, skinny, vanilla, extra hot, no foam latte right before you go to bed. Basically, don't drink anything that has any caffeine in it. Don't order that drink. Period.

Caffeine, if you didn't know, is a type of stimulant. It's a drug. What do stimulants do? You guessed it! They stimulate, which is the exact opposite of what you want if you plan on getting a good night's rest. You don't need more energy; you need to relax and calm your mind.

4. Sleep Hacks If You Study/Work From Home

If you are somebody who has to spend time on your computer at night, consider installing an app like F.lux [15].

What does it do? It syncs with the sunrise and sunset in your time zone, gradually shifting your screen's hue from blue and bright to red and dim.

Your screen is going to look a little weird at first, but you get used to it pretty fast. It's definitely a game changer in terms of being able to use your computer at night without it affecting your sleep.

Also, if you find yourself getting lost on Facebook or Twitter at some ungodly hour every night, you can use apps that block you from those sites at certain times, like the self-control app [16].

Something I've found very useful is installing an app on my phone called Sleep Cycle. It's available for both Android and iPhone users. You simply put the time when you want to wake up and put your phone on your bed or your nightstand. The app will wake you up from the lightest phase of sleep, which is your natural waking point. Because it also tracks your sleep incredibly accurately, it's the best 99 cents I've ever spent—next to all the five-cent candies I used to buy when I was a kid.

In a perfect world, you want to avoid electronic screens for at least an hour before going to bed. I know most of us use social media as a way to kill time before we go to sleep, but there are plenty of other things you can do that don't involve sticking your phone to your face.

You can read a book. When was the last time you started and finished one? You can journal about your day or you can meditate.

5. Practice Mindfulness

Practicing mindfulness through meditation is one of the best things you can do if you're one of those people with endless thoughts running through your head at night. It's the best way to bring you back to the moment, and it forces you to be as present as humanly possible.

If you're one of those people with some resistance to practicing meditation, it's nothing more than just finding a small window of your time when you simply focus on your breathing and just be in the moment.

It sounds so stupidly simple, but it's one of the most effective things you can do for yourself. You can download free apps like Calm, Headspace, and Insight Timer if you want to get started on guided meditation.

Set Yourself Up for Success

Do you ever get good sleep in an uncomfortable bed? Me neither.

You want to make sure you sleep in a comfortable bed. It blows my mind when people overlook this part.

If you often wake up with a sore back or an aching neck, you might want to think about investing in a new mattress, a new pillow, or both.

According to the trusty Sleep Country website, if your mattress is seven or more years old, a new mattress will likely improve your sleep.

If you're still using the same mattress from back when you were in high school, then it might be time to start thinking about buying a new one.

Time Your Workouts

Quick note on working out. I love it. I'm all for it. There's gonna be a separate chapter later on dedicated solely to this topic.

Working out during the day or doing something physically active can help you fall asleep faster at night because your body needs to recover from the stress you just put it through.

Just make sure you're not doing sprints minutes before you have to go to bed. Your heart rate is increased every time you work out, and you have to give your body a chance to cool down a little bit.

Remember, sleep is not an option. Don't worry about getting everything perfect right away. I'm not expecting a complete overnight bedroom makeover here. Change one or two things about your current sleeping strategy and go from there.

Again, this can all be done very quickly. If you mess up, just try to do better the next day. It might not seem like much, but this is the part you want to get right first and foremost.

Ignore it and it's going to be an uphill battle moving forward.

ACTION STEPS

Pick one of the sleep hacks I showed you and try it out tonight, whether that's setting your phone to *do not disturb* or airplane mode, using a sleep mask, or trying out the Sleep Cycle app. Just pick one. Again, don't worry about being perfect right away. Just be good.

Part 3: Nutrition

"A lot of people will do a lot of things to lose weight, except eat less and exercise." – Carlo Macapinlac
Yes, I just quoted myself.

Chapter 6: Do Not Read Another Fitness Article Until You Read This

Sometimes less is more.

Let me explain.

I'm sure you've heard the saying "knowledge is power" once or twice in your life, and for the most part, I agree with it.

You want to make sure your doctor has all the right information before he operates on you. You want your lawyer to be able argue your case properly. You want your engineer to have all the right numbers.

But we also know a person who's on his eighth year of university and has acquired multiple degrees. This person has also read more books in a month than you have in your entire life.

There's only one problem: they have nothing to show for all the information they've collected.

Then there are those college dropouts who only knew one thing. But they had a clear vision for what they wanted to do, got in the trenches, and are now retired and lying on a tropical beach somewhere.

I believe that there are two types of people in this world: there are researchers and there are go-getters.

Somewhere between the two is where you want to be. Bruce Lee said it best: "I fear not the man who has practiced 10,000 kicks once, but I fear the man who has practiced one kick 10,000 times."

You want to arm yourself with all the right tools in your toolbox and acquire as much information as you possibly can in order to give yourself the best chance to succeed.

This is when you put your "researcher" hat on.

More knowledge is rarely a bad thing, but there comes a time when you have to switch hats and translate all your knowledge into action. This is when you flip the switch and become a go-getter.

The problem is, most people get stuck on research mode.

Why? Because it's comfortable. It's easy. When you acquire new information, it makes you feel good. It almost gives you this feeling that you've already done the work, and this can be a very dangerous thing.

Think about the last time you read the latest revolutionary diet or weight loss article promising you fast and easy results. You get excited. You've already thought about all the things you're gonna do, all the new clothes you're gonna buy, and all the pool parties you're gonna attend because you just can't wait to take your shirt off and show your new and improved body to the world.

The next day, you find an even better weight loss strategy from a magazine promising even crazier results. So you do a little bit more research about this strategy. Then the next day comes and you're slapped again with a new diet and more information, and you go on and on until the entire thing turns into a vicious cycle.

You're stuck in research purgatory.

If you're one of those people who believe that consuming more information and waiting for the right opportunity will somehow set you up for better success, you probably suffer from something I like to call paralysis by analysis.

It's a condition where we're always trying to acquire more knowledge about a certain subject, thinking it will make us better. But the exact opposite ends up happening, and it delays us from taking action. It can be downright paralyzing because you keep getting high from doing research because it feels good.

You can look up all the variations on how to do a proper push-up or how to do a bench press, but if you don't take action, you're still gonna be stuck at zero.

There will never be a perfect moment or opportunity to do something. Nike was right when they said "Just Do It."

I'm also gonna mention this now so it doesn't come as a surprise to you. You're probably gonna mess up once or twice along the way. Nobody gets it right the first time.

And that's okay.

When it comes to reaching your goals, taking action is what actually moves the needle, not that shiny new fitness article you read while waiting to pay for your groceries.

Just remember that done is better than perfect.

The next chapter might be a reality check for some people reading this book, but bear with me on it. It's all going to make sense at the end.

Chapter 7: The Real Reason Why Your Last Diet Didn't Work

You've tried it all.

You've gone Paleo. You skipped eating fat. You ate more protein. You drank lemonade mixed with cayenne pepper. You tried drinking $10 cold-pressed juice. You tried "freezing" away your fat. You even experimented with going vegan.

You've tried spinning. You danced your butt off doing Zumba. You've done about a million sit-ups. You bought P90X. You even tried kickboxing.

Unfortunately, none of it worked.

I could spend the rest of this book trying to explain why you didn't get the results you were looking for, but I've found there's really only one common denominator in all of this.

Your attitude.

This is something I talk about a lot throughout this book—but for good reason. If you have a shitty attitude, you're not gonna get results. Period.

You could have the best diet and the best workout program, but if you have a terrible attitude and you're not willing to put in the work, you might as well not even try.

You need to stop complaining about how hard you have it and how difficult your life is. Stop playing the victim card.

Why? Because there are people out there who *really* have it rough.

People are getting their homes bombed. Have you seen the news lately? They have nothing to eat. The last thing they're complaining about is why the coffee shop is out of soy milk. Some people are born with disabilities. Some people get into car accidents and get limbs taken away from them. They're the ones who have it rough.

If you have a roof over your head, have food on the table, have a job, can use both your arms and legs, have a cell phone, and have time to go on social media and watch dog videos or whatever you're into, then you really don't have much to complain about.

If you have access to clean drinking water, you are among the luckiest of all humans on earth. Yet you'll always find an endless list of people complaining about pretty much anything and everything under the sun.

People complain about the weather. People complain about how hard it is not to eat chips while watching TV. They complain about how it's hard to resist popcorn when they go to the theater.

People complain about how hard it is to motivate them-selves to work out after a long day at work and how they have no time to pay attention to their diet. Yet these are the same people who watch hours and hours of Netflix every night.

People complain about how it's so hard to lose weight. Yet these are the same people who are first at the buffet line.

They say you can tell the size of a person by the size of the thing that bothers him.

Your attitude toward anything will determine your out-come. You can always control it. I want you to take a minute to put into perspective the majority of your problems and issues and your attitude toward them.

It's too hard to work out. Think about quadriplegic people who would probably give up just about any-thing if there was even a chance they could take a sin-gle step again.

You're complaining about eating leftovers. Think about homeless people going through dumpsters right now, looking for something to eat.

You're writing a list of things you want to change as part of your New Year's resolution, so you just delay everything until then. The thing is, life shouldn't start on January 1.

Stop waiting for the right opportunity. There will never be a perfect moment.

Yes, it's going to be *hard*. It took you months, even years, to get to your current state. Why would you expect things to just change overnight?

Listen, we're all given the same 24 hours. If you spend your time doing half-assed work, you're going to live a half-assed life.

Anything worth having takes time. If you're going to do something, you need to fully commit to it. Don't just do it when it's convenient for you.

Chapter 8: Breakfast Is the Biggest Con of Your Life

We've all seen it.

One commercial after another advertising breakfast cereals and granola bars to be a healthy way to start your day. And hey, don't forget to drink your glass of orange juice to get your daily dose of vitamin C!

Cereal packaging is even branded to be low in fat and fortified with vitamins and minerals. It even lists health claims like how it "contains whole grains."

So magically, people run to the grocery store to buy this stuff. We naturally think it must be good for us.

Breakfast is the most important meal of the day, right? Right??

The problem is, the "healthiest" low-fat options out there, and breakfast in general, might be one of the worst offenders when it comes to sabotaging your health.

Why "Fat-Free" Food Is Making You Fat

Let's use breakfast cereals as an example. It's a breakfast staple for a lot of people. Half a cup of low-fat granola, which is around 49 grams, contains 14 grams of sugar [17].

Even when that's all fine and well, nobody eats just half a cup of cereal! Most of the time, we just open the box, dump this stuff in a bowl, and go to town until we finish it.

Other research found that many low-fat foods marketed as "healthier" options contained *more* sugar than their full-fat equivalents [18]. There's got to be a way to make them "fat-free," right? That usually means adding sugar. Lots of it.

Many people associate the term "low-fat" as being healthy food. It turns out that statement is pretty inaccurate.

Breakfast cereals also make an appearance as an on-the-go snack in the form of a granola bar or "energy bar." It's a very popular snack for busy people because it's convenient and easy to consume.

The problem is, most cereals/granola bars are loaded with sugar! You're basically eating a glorified Snickers bar!

If you look on the back of the label, most of these bars are made with high-fructose corn syrup.

Why is this bad?

Excess amounts of fructose have been linked to increased risk of obesity, heart disease, kidney disease, type 2 diabetes, and other health problems [19].

You just don't want to be consuming this stuff in large amounts. Just because it's labeled "fat-free" doesn't mean it gets a free pass and it's automatically good for you. Learn to read the nutrition facts before you put anything in your mouth.

Long story short, just don't be one of those people that thinks substituting everything for low-fat food is automatically better for you. Fat doesn't make you fat. Overeating does.

Orange Juice Is the Enemy

Think about the usual suspects for your typical breakfast back when you were a kid or even until now.

You've got your favorite breakfast cereal, maybe some eggs, bacon, and some toast, or maybe even a combination of all four. But there was always one thing that made a consistent appearance. We were always served a glass (or two) of orange juice.

Truth be told, I never really questioned it. It's part of a complete breakfast, right? After all, you need your daily dose of vitamin C.

The problem is, if we look at its nutritional profile, orange juice isn't much better than Coke, Gatorade, or any other sweetened drink that's being marketed right now.

Yet the latter get demonized, for fair reasons, and the former seems to get a pass.

Does it have vitamins and minerals? Sure! But there are far better ways to get your daily vitamins than drinking orange juice. A balanced diet of vegetables, fruits, nuts, and grains would be a good place to start.

Vegetables like broccoli, bell pepper, dark leafy greens, and tomatoes contain high amounts of vitamin C if you're looking for some alternatives when it comes to getting your daily dose.

The problem with drinking orange juice or any other types of juice for that matter is that one key thing gets removed during the juice extraction process: fiber.

Fiber is one of the key factors when it comes to helping you feel full and satisfied until your next meal. In short, it prevents you from overeating. If you take fiber out of the fruit, you're left with sugar, water, and vitamin C. You're basically drinking Gatorade.

A typical 12-ounce glass of orange juice contains around 10 oranges. The problem is, who the hell eats 10 oranges in one sitting? The serving size is just way too much.

Here's the nutritional profile for a 12-ounce glass of orange juice [20]:

153 calories

35.38 grams of carbohydrates

28.58 grams of sugar

2.38 grams of protein

0.7 grams of dietary fiber

That's the same number of carbs and just three grams less sugar than a bag of M&M's [21]. Yet we drink orange juice like it's going out of style and we treat a bag of M&M's as the second coming of the devil.

At the end of the day, it's all about taking responsibility for what you're putting in your body. Specifically, that means knowing the right serving size and not just mindlessly consuming things because society told you it's okay to do so.

Chapter 9: One Step Back, Two Steps Forward

"You must unlearn what you have learned." – Master Yoda

Before we go any further, we need a clean slate. I want you to wipe everything that you've learned about diet and nutrition so far and start clean.

Just like the rest of this page.

There's just so much misleading and garbage information out there, so let's throw all that out the window and give you the cold, hard truth about how everything works. No weight loss tea, no diet pills, and no weight loss straps. And no, we're not gonna "freeze" your fat away.

Just to be clear, I'm not a doctor, dietician, or nutritionist. I am an educated trainer, a national-level weightlifter, and a health and fitness coach. What I'm going to share with you is a two-pronged approach to eating that I've perfected through years of trial and error, and it has literally changed my life and the lives of my students.

It's a replicable system you can use to get real, sustainable, long-lasting results that you can maintain as long as you want to stay healthy and fit.

Now raise your hand if you've ever tried a detox, a cleanse, a weight loss pill, or a weight loss strap that you bought from a TV infomercial, or maybe your friend told you about the next revolutionary diet claiming to be the be-all and end-all to your weight loss success?

Okay, you can put your hand down now.

Diets are awesome when you think about it. You get promised "fast" and "easy" results if you just follow X, Y, and Z. You read about the types of food you can and can't eat—like zero carbs, low fat, and low every-thing and drink concoctions such as juice cleanses and everything seems so easy.

I even saw an ad the other day about "freezing away" your fat. What. The. Hell.

But when it comes to execution and consistency of these aforementioned diets, that's when things start to fall apart.

For short periods of time—the key word here is *short*—every diet/cleanse will work if it puts you in some form of calorie restriction. Yay for instant re-sults, right?

But whether it's the lack of time to prepare those six small meals a day or the diet being too restrictive, you can't just drink weight loss tea for the rest of your life. It's too complicated in general (10 days of just drink-ing lemonade, no dairy, no gluten, no red meat, no carbs, no fat—basically just eating air), so you're bound to go back to your old habits once the diet is over. It's just not sustainable.

Ever heard of the show *The Biggest Loser*? It's inspir-ing to watch all the contestants go through their trans-formations, right? But there's an ugly side to it. Re-search of 14 of their contestants shows that, after six years, they gained back most of the weight they lost from the show [22].

How do I know these things? It's simple. I've been there before. I was *that* guy. Although I've never made it to *The Biggest Loser*, I've literally tried thousands of workouts and jumped around from diets and cleanses only to be disappointed every time because I didn't get the results I was promised.

It's just another example of putting a Band-Aid on a bigger problem. I struggled with this trial and error method for *years*, always looking for that quick fix, that get skinny fast method. I have some bad news for you. It doesn't work like that. It doesn't help that we live in a society that likes to treat the symptom rather than the problem itself.

There is no "right" way to eat. We all have different preferences when it comes to food. You can't just delete certain food groups from your diet, especially if it's the type of food you love, and expect it to last. We are human beings. We're conditioned to always want what we can't have. The more you tell someone they can't have ice-cream, the more they'll want to quit their diet and buy a tub of Ben & Jerry's cookie dough. On a serious note, have you tried that flavor? It'll change your life.

But what if I told you this type of restrictive and complicated diet is simply not necessary for weight loss? What if I told you there *is* a way to eat that can give you amazing health benefits, help you lose weight, and even build muscle *without* being restricted to any type of food?

I mean, who doesn't want to have a six pack? The best part is, it does not involve any prolonged periods of food restrictions, deleting entire food groups, crazy meal plans, or wearing silly-looking straps.

It turns out that it's not about what you eat—but when you eat.

Chapter 10: The "No Diet" Diet Approach to Eating

I haven't eaten breakfast since 2012.

What I mean by that is I don't eat first thing in the morning like 99% of the general population. Instead, I eat two big meals: one at 1:00 p.m. and I finish eating my second meal at 9:00 p.m. I might have a small snack in between those two big meals if I feel like it. The rest of the time, I don't worry about what I eat.

No, I'm not on any sort of revolutionary diet. What I do is a pattern of eating called **intermittent fasting**. It's a way of scheduling your meals so that you get the most out of them.

You don't have to change what you eat; you just have to change when you eat. Simple!

Again, let me repeat that because this is the base of everything in the next couple of chapters.

You don't have to change what you eat; you just have to change when you eat (and how much of it).

There, I just revealed to you the secret to life. Now go ahead and get shredded and live your best life. You can stop reading this book now. Just kidding. There's more to it than just fasting.

I first discovered intermittent fasting from a book called *Eat Stop Eat* by Brad Pilon, and I later adapted the lean gains method to intermittent fasting by Martin Berkhan. I didn't invent this stuff. I just adapted the method and made it my own. I just want to give credit where credit is due, so big high fives to Brad and Martin.

As mentioned earlier, intermittent fasting is not the be-all and end-all to weight loss. There's more to it than just taking a break from eating. To maximize my results, I started tracking my macros. I started paying attention to how much food I'm putting in my body. I use a free phone app called MyFitnessPal to do this, and it's been a complete game changer to my diet.

This is what allows me to still eat whatever I want. I just have to control the amount I'm consuming. No, I'm not saying you should weigh every ounce of food you eat every day. But it's a great practice if you're just starting out.

After a while, you'll have a general idea of how much food you should be eating, and at that point, you can just start going by feel. This is what I call "intuitive eating," and it comes from good daily practice until it becomes second nature. I've simplified my life even further by eating the same meal every day or a small variation of it. That way, I don't have to worry about what I'm going to eat.

Combining intuitive eating with intermittent fasting is what turned everything around for me. It's when real change started to happen. I started seeing results I've been able to maintain, and my body thrives from it. I still do it up to this day.

I'm not restricted to any type of food. I just control how much of it I consume in one sitting. Hence the "No Diet" Diet was born.

Here's the "No Diet" Diet summarized in one equation:

Intermittent Fasting + Tracking Your Macros = Lean Sexy Body

Here's some proof. Go to:

>>> http://www.newbiefitnessacademy.com/before-and-after

It's the same person in each picture but a completely different body, and they both lived completely different lives. Before you start freaking out that it's not the same person, the picture on the right was taken in front of a mirror—hence the inverted tattoo.

The guy on the left had low self-confidence. I hated how my body looked. If you look closely, I was using my bag to hide my belly. I binged on whatever was in front of me. I avoided every situation where I had to take my shirt off in public. I didn't have a lot of friends.

I bought baggy clothes to hide my dad bod. I was unhappy with my life.

The guy on the right lives his best life every day. He walks around as if he's five inches taller because he actually likes himself. He likes the way his body looks. He's a fierce weekend warrior. He has a lot of friends. Endless opportunities come to his life because he has a great relationship with himself, and it shows when he interacts with people.

Which person would you rather be?

Sometimes it's not about the weight you lose but about the life you gain.

I feel like I'm finally living the life that was robbed from me back in those years when I didn't have my health and fitness in check. I didn't know I was holding myself back from a life of abundance simply because I didn't have a good relationship with myself and it stemmed mostly from how I felt about my body.

Now let's talk about some cold, hard numbers. The first couple of months (eight weeks) of following the "No Diet" Diet, I went from 136 pounds to 121.8 pounds. That's just over a 14-pound weight loss. Now that might not sound like much, but that's a whopping 11% of my body weight.

Based on my experience with past students, your numbers could be even bigger if you have more fat to lose.

I'm not the biggest guy, after all. The best part is that I've been able to maintain my results and even add more muscle to my frame after six years of being on the "No Diet" Diet.

Keep in mind that I'm nothing special. I wasn't the popular quarterback in high school. I was never naturally good at sports. In fact, I ate Doritos in the stands while I watched our high school team do sports. I wasn't blessed with what you would call good genetics. I was always the chubby kid growing up, and now, I'm a national-level weightlifter.

In short, I'm just a regular guy who managed to put it all together. I mean, I only failed 43,261,543 times. But that's okay. I've already made all the mistakes so you don't have to.

Now you may be wondering.

You can get all of this from fasting? How is this possible?

What the hell are macros? Is it short for macaroni?

Isn't breakfast the most important meal of the day?

What are the benefits of doing this?

This is too good to be true! What's the catch?

I'm going to try my best to not bore you with useless data and statistics and make you feel like you're in high school biology again. I'll just give you cold, hard facts backed by research and my own personal experience.

By the end of this book, the only thing you're gonna ask yourself is, "When do I start?"

Chapter 11: What Is Intermittent Fasting and Why Should You Do It?

The short answer is because it works. Plain and simple.

The long answer is that intermittent fasting is an eating pattern where you switch between periods of eating and fasting. It doesn't have any rules about what type of food you have to eat, only *when* you should eat.

I want you to think of it as simply taking a break from eating when you're on a fast.

If we go back a little bit into history, you'll actually find that fasting has been around as early as the caveman days. Back then, fasting wasn't really by choice but a way of life as our hunting ancestors didn't really know when they were going to eat next until their next successful hunt. They also didn't have refrigerators to store their leftovers back then. They ate until their next meal was available.

A lot of religions, like Islam, incorporate fasting in their beliefs. Muslims fast every day from dawn to sunset for the entire month of Ramadan. Notice how your Muslim friends look a little leaner after this time? And they're not even doing it to lose weight.

This isn't some foreign thing that just came about recently. It's been around since the beginning of time and there's data and research to prove that it works.

The problem is, you can't sell fasting to make money.

It's bad for businesses because it simply doesn't move any product. Thus, we hear inaccurate statements like "breakfast is the most important meal of the day," "eat six small meals every day to increase your metabolism," "eat every three hours," "eat gluten-free," and "eat zero calorie/nonfat."

Basically, eat everything.

We're constantly being told what to eat in order to lose weight. It makes absolutely no sense.

I'm gonna borrow a quote from Brad Pilon from his book *Eat Stop Eat* because he does a great job of simplifying everything you need to know about nutrition. He said there are only two absolute facts when it comes to nutrition and weight loss:

1. Prolonged caloric restriction is the only proven nutritional method of weight loss.

2. Human beings can only be in one of the following states: fed or fasted.

That's it.

The way you view food and nutrition should revolve around those two facts. Everything else is just fluff in the clouds trying to sell you stuff that you don't need.

Let's dive into those two facts a little bit more.

1) Prolonged caloric restriction is the only proven nutritional method of weight loss

You simply can't lose weight if you're always constantly eating. I know, mind-blowing stuff, right?

Yet we spend all day thinking about what to eat, preparing, eating, and cleaning up. Then you repeat that cycle again a couple of hours later for the next meal. We basically spend all day thinking about what we're going to eat next.

As mentioned earlier, the problem with fasting is that it's not a very marketable topic. There's nothing sexy about it. It's hard to lose weight and get the body you want when all you're told is that you need to eat more. In a world full of fancy diets with endless features and highlights, it goes the complete opposite way by telling you to simply take a break from eating.

People can't seem to grasp that simple idea because it's been ingrained in our heads that we need to be eating all the time.

The Definition of Fasting

Let's quickly define the word *fasting* because there seems to be a lot of negative stigma surrounding this word popularized by nothing but bro-science and cooler talk.

This is pulled right out of dictionary.com. Their definition of fasting is as follows: "An abstinence from food, or a limiting of one's food, especially when voluntary and as a religious observance" [23].

Let's focus on one key word in that statement: *voluntary*. That's the biggest difference between fasting and starving. In case you really need to know, you don't enter starvation mode until about 96 hours or longer without food.

You'd actually be shocked how long your body can function without food, as long as you're properly hydrated. Forty-eight hours? No problem. Twenty-four hours? Piece of cake. But I'm not even asking for that. I'm only asking for a 16-hour fast or basically just skipping breakfast. That's it.

Taking a short break from eating equals awesome results. That's not a bad trade-off if you ask me.

2) Human beings can only be in one of the following states: fed or fasted.

Fed State – Any time you're putting food in your mouth.

Fasted State – After you're done eating, that's when your fast starts and your body slowly transitions to the fasted state. Once your body is done digesting the food in your stomach, that's when it starts to use body fat as a source of energy.

Translation? Your body literally starts to become a fat-burning machine during the fasted state. You start getting the full effects of this crazy phenomenon 16–24 hours after your last meal.

That's how the 16-hour fast was born. Do this every day and watch your body transform right before your very eyes.

The problem is that we've been trained to eat as many as six meals a day by today's society, so we're always in the fed state. We're constantly eating food to "lose weight."

It just doesn't make sense. We're always in fat-storage mode instead of giving our bodies a chance to turn into fat-burning mode, and that again only happens when we're in the fasted state.

You're Already Doing It

I'm going to tell you something that will blow your mind.

All of us already fast every single day—it's called sleeping. Intermittent fasting just means extending that fasting period for a few more hours.

For example, let's say you finish eating dinner at 7:00 p.m. Your body will then begin to slowly switch from the fed to the fasted state. You go to bed and you simply skip breakfast the next day. For this example, you complete the 16-hour fast at 11:00 a.m.

That's it. You're only skipping one meal. If somebody told me before that I'm gonna get all the results I've always wanted, and then some, by simply taking a break from eating, I would've started a long time ago.

Fasting Myths Debunked

The amount of anti-fasting information that can be found on the Internet is pretty staggering. In a world where we're constantly told what to eat in order to lose weight, it's almost taboo to say it can be as simple as not eating for a certain period of time.

Think about the last time you got your blood tested. Your doctor said you needed to be fasted until blood was taken. Perfectly normal, right?

But to use fasting as a way to lose weight? Blasphemy.

It's usually then followed up by ridiculous statements such as "Fasting kills your metabolism," "The weight you lose is all muscle," or "I would die if I fasted." This is typical of fasting misinformation.

Add in the fact that we've been told since the beginning of time that "breakfast is the most important meal of the day" or that "you need to eat six small meals a day."

This is an example of authoritative parroting where people simply repeat what they've heard from "experts" on the topic without actually stopping to check and see if what they've heard is correct. So the same misinformation is repeated, whether it's accurate or not, until it becomes the truth.

For the rest of this chapter, I'm going to play the role of *MythBusters* and debunk some of the most popular myths about fasting and just give you the cold, hard facts once and for all.

Myth #1: "Fasting will *kill* your metabolism."

You're gonna hear that statement a lot when you start fasting, but nothing could be further from the truth. Wikipedia defines the word metabolism, also known as your basal metabolic rate (BMR), as "The amount of energy per unit time that a person needs to keep the body functioning at rest" [24].

It's the amount of energy needed just to be you. The average BMR for men is between 1600 and 2000 calories [25]. That number could be higher depending on your height and weight, but let's use 2000 calories as an example.

Your body will always burn 2000 calories, even if you just sit on the couch all day and watch paint dry. If you decide to move around and exercise, the calories you burn from working out are just always added to your BMR.

So why have we been led to believe that fasting will kill your metabolism and been told to eat six small meals a day to "boost" your metabolism?

This just goes back to food advertising and giant corporations selling you breakfast cereals and meal replacement bars or whatever new product they're currently promoting.

According to **research** from 2012, restaurants spent almost $6 billion just on advertising alone in the United States [26]. McDonald's takes the cake in the category, spending almost $1 billion. No wonder Americans can't get enough of their Big Macs.

Think of all the companies that would go under if they spent their advertising dollars telling you not to buy their products and just fast. They would all go bankrupt. Instead, it's ingrained in our heads that we need to buy more and eat more meals.

In fact, one study shows that eating more frequently does absolutely nothing for your weight loss and metabolic rate [27]. Again, how could you possibly lose weight by always eating? *It makes no sense.*

Your BMR stays the same no matter what. That is a fact. It's just bro-science if they tell you otherwise.

And lastly, another study shows that you can fast for 72 hours and not see any changes in your metabolism [28]. I wouldn't recommend fasting that long, but you get the point. Your metabolism won't go haywire if you fast.

Myth #2: "You'll lose muscle mass when you fast."

You'll often hear other ridiculous statements in conjunction with this myth, like "You should never exercise on an empty stomach" or "Fasted training will burn your muscles."

Based on research by Proeyen et al., that myth is completely inaccurate [29]. Studies have found that working out while fasted (aka fasted training) is actually a great way to build muscle mass, is great for fat loss, and can even boost insulin sensitivity [30–32].

Now here's the good stuff.

When you fast, the growth hormone response is triggered, and this is what prevents people from losing muscle. A five-day study of six perfectly healthy male adults revealed that human growth hormone levels were as high as 2000% from the baseline right at the 24-hour mark of the first day [33].

Not 200%: 2000%! That's insane! That's like taking steroids without all the bad side effects. And it's free!

Not only does fasting *not* slow down your metabolism, but it also doesn't result in your body devouring your muscles. Your body is designed to fast.

There's only one catch in order to prove this myth wrong. You have to be involved in some form of resistance training to maintain your hard-earned muscles. Unfortunately, there's no something-for-nothing deal here.

Think of people in hospital beds, for example. They're involved in some form of caloric restriction while they're confined to the hospital, but because they're not able to exercise, they start to lose muscle mass.

Intermittent fasting works, but it's not a magic pill. You can't just magically expect to hold onto your muscles if you're not working out. There's no free lunch here.

Myth #3: "I would die if I fast."

This is probably my favorite myth to debunk because it shows exactly the unhealthy relationship we've developed when it comes to food.

Short answer: no, you won't die if you fast.

We as a society have developed a bad relationship with food over time. It's ingrained in our heads that we need to eat and drink all the time. We've turned into what I like to call "emotional eaters."

Think about it. What's the first thing we do when we're bored? What's the first thing we do when we're sad? What's the first thing we do when we see someone we haven't seen in a while?

We eat.

That's all fine and good. The problem is, we do it way too much. We're now using food as a form of entertainment and we need to be entertained all the time.

For the record, you'd have to go three weeks without eating anything before you actually died. Gandhi actually proved this when he went 21 days of complete starvation, and even he didn't die. Skipping breakfast and eating a late lunch is nothing compared to that.

Instead of viewing food as a source of fuel and nutrition to power you through everyday life, we've developed a habit of eating for pleasure instead. How many times have you caught yourself bored and the first thing you do is stuff food in your mouth so you have something to do?

Now I'm not against eating out—I think it's delicious. But how many times do you hear people plan their day around activities like going for lunch or dinner?

Why do we do this? Because it's easy. It's convenient. As mentioned earlier, it doesn't help that billions of dollars every year are used just on food marketing and advertising alone. No wonder eating is the first choice of activity for a lot of people!

We make as many as 200 decisions related to food alone every day. Every day! I don't know about you, but that sounds like a lot. Too many in fact. Your brain power can only process so much, and food shouldn't be your priority every single time. There are other pleasurable things in life besides just eating.

Long story short, our relationship with food is just something we've been accustomed to through our culture and surroundings. But if you want real change, you're gonna have to start thinking differently. You need to zig when everyone else zags, if you catch my drift.

I'm not saying that food is bad. I'm just saying that you need to learn how to control your urges when it comes to it. You have to learn how to say no to yourself every once in a while.

When you start doing intermittent fasting, you're gonna realize how much brain power you spend on food decisions alone, and you're gonna feel empowered to finally be in control.

You can't always let your urges control your decisions. Be stronger than your strongest excuse. It's a great feeling to know that, during your fast, you don't have to think about your next meal and you can start focusing on things that really matter.

Myth #4: "Breakfast is the most important meal of the day."

This is probably one of my favorites because it's one of the most popular myths out there. It's the kind of stuff that's been force fed to us since we were kids.

Short answer: no, breakfast isn't the most important meal of the day.

Let's talk about the meaning of the word *breakfast*. It's derived from the term *breaking fast*. When you eat breakfast, you're simply breaking your fast from your sleep the night before. We've just been led to believe that we need to do it first thing in the morning.

The thing is, you can break your fast anytime you want, meaning you can have your "breakfast" after you've completed your 16-hour fast. For example, I eat my "breakfast" at 1:00 p.m. every day.

The other thing is that if your breakfast involves a combination of pancakes with syrup, waffles with whipped cream, bacon, sausage, hash browns, breakfast sandwiches, a glass of orange juice, and a side of Baileys and coffee, that doesn't really sound like the most important meal of the day. It sounds more like the worst meal of the day. If you somehow skipped the first half of this book, there's an entire chapter dedicated to eating breakfast (see Chapter 8).

There's also no **scientific data** out there that says eating six small meals is somehow more beneficial for you than skipping your classic breakfast and just eating your meals in an eight-hour window [34]. As mentioned earlier, $8 billion is spent every year to make us believe that we need to eat *all the time*.

Listen, I love food just as much as the next guy. All I'm saying is that it's okay to take a break from it every once in a while and let our body's natural fat-burning mechanism do the work for us.

Chapter 12: The Benefits of Taking a Break from Eating

Any diet will work if it puts you in some form of caloric restriction.

That's why it's easy for people to fall in love with juice cleanses. Add the big T-word—toxins—into the equation, and people line up for a seven-day juice cleanse package for $299 like it's going out of style. Who pays $299 for juice anyway??

Fear can be a very powerful thing when it comes to advertising. When you're led to believe that there's these little demons living inside you, eating you away from the inside, it's game over.

But what happens after you're done your juice cleanse? You simply go back to your old habits until you feel like you need to get rid of the built-up toxins in your body again. That'll be another $299, please.

People don't really fail with diets. They fail to maintain them. It's hard to live off liquid calories or delete entire food groups, like the Ketogenic diet, for the rest of your life.

One of the biggest reasons why intermittent fasting is a more sustainable way of eating versus dieting is because it's easy to maintain. You don't always have to think about what to eat for breakfast every day. You don't always have to bring a small Tupperware everywhere you go so you can eat your small meal every three hours.

The crazy part is that there are other cool things that only get activated in your body when you take a break from eating. It turns out that weight loss is just the tip of the iceberg. Let's dive in a little deeper and talk about some of the other awesome changes that occur in your body during your fast.

How to Fight Diabetes

According to research, as of 2015, 30.3 million Americans, or 9.4% of the U.S. population, have diabetes [35]. That's one in every 10, which is pretty staggering. It's the seventh leading cause of death in America. I can't imagine that number being any lower right now.

Type 2 diabetes occurs when the pancreas doesn't make enough insulin or the body does not use insulin properly. This is called insulin resistance. As a result, glucose—a simple sugar that's an important energy source—can't be moved from the blood and into the body's cells.

Insulin is one of the most important hormones in your body. It helps keep your blood sugar levels from getting too high or too low. I don't want to turn this book into Biology 101, but one quick Google search and you'll find out why insulin is crucial to your health.

Whenever you eat, your blood insulin levels increase. The increased amount of insulin drives the storage of nutrients within your body. This function is important to keep you alive. So far so good, right?

When insulin levels are high, you are in fat storage mode. Plain and simple. The key idea to remember is when your insulin is high, your body fat isn't going anywhere. Are you with me so far?

The problem starts with the fact that we are simply eating too much too often. Six small meals, anyone? As a result, we're always in fat storage mode because our insulin levels are always elevated. The bigger issue is, chronically elevated insulin levels are associated with the development of insulin resistance, diabetes, and other forms of disease.

This is where intermittent fasting comes to the rescue. In a study by Barnosky et al., blood sugar was reduced by 3–6% while fasting, and insulin dropped by 20–31% [36].

Once you switch from the fed state to the fasted state, blood levels of insulin drop significantly, which activates the natural fat-burning mechanism in your body [37].

By simply taking a break from eating, you create small periods of time when insulin levels are allowed to become very low. This is when your body turns fat into a source of energy. Combine this with sensible eating, and you're setting yourself up for long-term health while protecting yourself from the risk of developing type 2 diabetes.

How to Boost Your Testosterone and Growth Hormones for Free

Multiple studies [38] show that every time you eat something, your testosterone levels drop. If you're a man, I probably don't need to explain to you why that's important.

Eating breakfast first thing in the morning and consuming multiple small meals throughout the day would only plummet your testosterone levels even more with every meal. Yet these are things that get advertised to be a good thing every day.

Crazy.

Your growth hormone levels also go down every time your insulin level goes up. Think of it as a lever [39]. So if you eat your six small meals during the day, then you also get an insulin spike six times a day, which means you're in fat storage mode all day. Your growth hormone levels and testosterone also plummet multiple times a day. Not a good combination at all.

Here's where it gets interesting. A study on healthy, non-obese single guys noted an amazing 180% increase in testosterone levels, just from short periods of fasting [40], meaning that intermittent fasting will have an instant positive effect on your testosterone levels.

Testosterone levels are actually highest in the morning [41], and it just happens to coincide with an overnight fast—also called sleeping.

In a study by Ho et al., researchers saw that after 24 hours of consuming no calories, growth hormone levels were elevated 2000% from the baseline [42]. Not 200% but 2000%. Long story short, intermittent fasting is one of the best tools you could use to increase your natural testosterone and growth hormone production.

You hear this a lot in sports, mainly about athletes injecting themselves with synthetic testosterone and human growth hormones because it's easily the fastest way to gain lean muscle mass, which increases strength while simultaneously burning fat in a short period of time. It also increases healing rate, which is important for training and maintaining peak performance.

However, these banned substances create a vast list of side effects when taken in synthetic, unnatural forms. So we're just gonna say no to that stuff.

Most people believe that you can't have a significant increase in either one of those hormones without the use of injections or steroids. It turns out that all you have to do is take a break from eating. And it's free!

There's not many things that can give you a nice 180% increase in testosterone and a 2000% increase in growth hormones from the baseline as quickly as just one day of intermittent fasting can.

The Best Cleanse on the Planet

Toxins.

The big scary T-word. As mentioned earlier, we live in a society where that word gets thrown around by everyone like it's Halloween candy. They're bad for us. We need to get rid of them or they'll eat us away from the inside.

Our solution? Juice cleanses and detox diets.

The thing is, we don't need to go on those crazy liquid diets. Our bodies get rid of harmful toxins all on their own—regardless of how much $10 kale ginger celery carrot beet cold-pressed juice you drink. That'll be another $299, please.

Forget about drinking your weight in juice to flush out toxins. There's a free and easier way to do it. Also, I'm starting to think that I should've priced this book at $299 instead of $2.99. I'm basically like a juicing company, minus the juice. Now I'm starting to think that I should start a juicing company.

The good news: there's a little-known way your body *does* cleanse itself, and it's a process you can control. You just need to do some self-cannibalism.

What?

No, I'm not asking you to eat your own fingers to prevent yourself from putting crap in your body. Although, that's another way of doing it.

I'm talking about self-cannibalism on a cellular level called autophagy [43]. The word literally means "eating of self."

Autophagy is a form of cellular maintenance or cleansing. In the simplest of terms, it's our body's natural system of cleaning house. Your body hunts for dead, diseased, or worn-out cells and replaces those damaged components with new ones within your body.

According to Colin Champ, MD and author of *Misguided Medicine*, "Autophagy makes us more efficient machines to get rid of faulty parts, stop cancerous growths, and stop metabolic dysfunction like obesity and diabetes" [44].

Your body literally flushes out everything it doesn't need. It's like "detox" on steroids.

How do we activate this process? You guessed it—through fasting [45]. What turns it off? You guessed right again—eating!

The more time you spend in the fed state, the less time you have to ramp up the autophagic process within your body. And they say that eating every three hours was good for you? At some point you gotta start asking yourself who comes up with these things.

This might be the mother of all benefits of intermittent fasting. Other than weight loss and boosting your testosterone and growth hormone levels, this might be the next best reason why you should take a break from eating.

The Fountain of Youth

A study on fasting from 1945 found that varying numbers of 24-hour fasts prolonged the lifespan of rats [46]. In one of the experiments, rats that fasted every other day lived 83% longer than rats who weren't fasted [47].

Another study showed that after only 16 weeks of eating the same food but in restricted fasting windows, mice had a 33% lower risk for certain cancer types [48,49].

The most likely explanation for this, which would indicate a similar benefit in humans, is the autophagic process I mentioned earlier. Autophagy gives your body a chance to get rid of cancerous cells and replace them with new ones.

If somebody told you there's something you can do to reduce the negative effects of aging [50], maintain muscle mass, increase testosterone production, and possibly even prevent cancer, Alzheimer's, and other types of disease, wouldn't you at least be compelled to try it? The fountain of youth might actually exist after all.

Chapter 13: Two Methods of Intermittent Fasting

I'm sure you're ready to try intermittent fasting at this point so let's talk about two of my preferred methods of doing it. As mentioned earlier, you get its full effects 16–24 hours after your last meal. Both methods that I'm about to show you fall within that range and are equally effective. Just pick one that suits your lifestyle the best.

The 24-Hour Fast

This method was popularized by Brad Pilon from his book *Eat Stop Eat* [51]. The main idea is to do a 24-hour fast once or twice a week.

Here's an example.

Let's say you have a 9:00 to 5:00 desk job. You get home from work and you finally get to finish eating dinner at 8:00 p.m. after taking care of all your errands. That's when your fast officially starts. You go to bed, and you simply skip breakfast and lunch the next day and you break your fast at 8:00 p.m. This is called a dinner-to-dinner fast. You can also do a lunch-to-lunch fast if that suits your lifestyle better. You're technically not going a full day without food. You're simply skipping two meals.

This is actually the first method of intermittent fasting I tried. I love it because you only have to do it once or twice a week. The rest of the time, you can eat your regular three meals per day. It's perfect if you're someone who really likes to eat first thing in the morning (i.e., if you have kids and you have to eat breakfast with them).

Just remember to leave 48 hours in between your fasts to let your body balance out your hormones. Yes, there is such a thing as too much of a good thing. You still need to eat. I'm just asking you to take a break from it.

The 16-Hour Fast

This is the method I follow to this day. This method is more popularly known as the lean gains method, and it was created by Martin Berkhan [52].

The main idea is to do a 16-hour fast every day. You then have an eight-hour "feeding" window to fulfill your daily macros allowance. More on this topic in the next chapter. You can eat two big meals or you can split up your daily calorie allowance into two smaller meals and a snack. It's up to you.

The key for both methods is flexibility. Try it out and see what works best for you.

4 Tips for Starting Your First Fast

Slow and steady wins the race. They say that it actually takes 66 days to make or break a habit, not the 21 days that we've been led to believe. If you've never fasted a day in your life before, start slow.

You don't have to go all or nothing here right away. You can simply start by just going 12 hours in the first week. Remember, our bodies are well equipped to handle fasting but it takes our minds a little bit longer to adjust to the process, especially when we've been so accustomed to eating all the time.

The following week, try extending it to 14 hours. Get some small victories under your belt. Then start ramping it up to 16 hours once you're more comfortable with it. Trust me, you'll barely feel the difference.

Stay hydrated. Staying well hydrated will make your fasting periods much easier to get through. Plus, our bodies are made up of 60% water, so you should be drinking plenty of this stuff anyway. To add variety, feel free to drink tea or black coffee during the fast.

The key is to drink stuff that has zero calories. I personally prefer tea, and there's enough variety of this stuff to keep things interesting. Also, try to avoid any zero-calorie soda. I'm just not a big fan of pop, and the number of chemicals that you and I can't even pronounce in these drinks to make them "zero calorie" is not worth the trouble.

Change your vocabulary. As mentioned earlier, think of fasting as simply taking a short break from eating, not as a period of starvation. This simple shift in your mind is one of the—if not *the* biggest—keys when it comes to changing your thoughts and behavior throughout this process.

Stay busy. You're going to be shocked by how much time taking small breaks from eating actually frees up. I don't know what your personal interests are, so I'm not gonna tell you what to do with your free time. But try to stay as busy as possible. This helps time pass. You can work out, you can get more work done at the office, you can read a book, you can walk your dog, or you can walk your neighbor's dog. Just do something other than thinking about your next meal.

Follow the 50/25/25 rule. Bonus tip. I'm all about giving away full value in this book. I don't believe in crazy diets but I believe in portion control. A good rule of thumb to follow is the 50/25/25 rule. Half your plate should consist of vegetables. While the other half should consist of carbs and protein. If you follow this rule, a plate of pasta with a side of toast might not be the most balanced meal after all.

Note: The 50/25/25 rule is part of the Ultimate Diet Hack Cheatsheet. The cheatsheet reveals nine quick ways to mindlessly hack your diet. Think of it as jedi mind tricks to your diet. To download your free copy, just go to:

>>> www.newbiefitnessacademy.com/diet-hack-cheatsheet

Final Thoughts About Fasting

You should check with your doctor before trying anything new. Fasting is considered safe in most cases but you shouldn't do it if the following apply to you.

You're pregnant. There's a human being growing inside of you. You should probably eat.

You have a history of eating disorder. I'm not a nutrition expert, but fasting might not be a good idea if your relationship with food is something you're struggling with.

You are chronically stressed. Short-term stress like fasting and exercise is good for our bodies and can have great benefits if done properly. But if you're someone who deals with a lot of stress at work and at home, then adding more stress to your life like fasting and exercise might be something you want to hold off.

You don't plan on working out. As mentioned earlier, being involved in some form of resistance training is how we hold onto our dear muscles when we fast. If you fast and don't exercise, you're going to lose both fat *and* muscle.

Fasting for Women

If you're following the 16-hour fast, according to LeanGains.com, women should start small with a 14 hour fast and eventually transition to 16 hours [53].

There's not a lot of benefit for women to do longer fasts, and a lot of it has to do with maintaining hormonal health. If you're a girl and you're reading this, just start with a 14-hour fast and see how your body responds.

If you plan on following the 24-hour fast method, then doing it once or twice a week should be perfectly safe.

ACTION STEPS

Pick your preferred method of fasting and try it out tomorrow. Remember to stay busy. Rinse and repeat. Now watch your body change right before your eyes.

Chapter 13: You Can't Control What You Can't Measure

The last couple of chapters were all about reframing our relationship with food. They talked about how it's okay to take a break from eating. It might even be the secret to fighting disease and achieving eternal youth. I also talked about my plan to start a juicing company, minus the juice.

This chapter is all about what to do when you actually eat—specifically, how to keep track of it.

Remember the "No Diet" Diet equation? Here it is again:

Intermittent Fasting + <u>Tracking Your Macros</u> = Lean Sexy Body

Ever heard of the 80/20 principle?

It's a crazy phenomenon because the entire world is subject to it. It was discovered by an Italian Economist named Vilfredo Pareto in the early 1900s when he realized that 80% of the wealth in Italy was held by 20% of the population.

But it was recently made much more popular by author Richard Koch. He realized that the 80/20 principle didn't just apply to wealth. It applied to *everything*.

20% of employees are responsible for 80% of the company's output.

20% of freeways get 80% of the traffic.

20% of customers make 80% of the purchases.

20% of runners win 80% of the races.

Long story short, most of the results of any situation are determined by a small number of causes. This is the 20% of work that will get you 80% of your results—maybe even 90%. It's that important. It's all about tracking your macros. Don't worry, it's not rocket science.

No, *macros* is not short for macaroni.

How to Track Your Macros

For a lot of people wanting to lose weight, it's easier to eat a little less than to move a little more. The problem is, we eat too much. If this is still news to you, you should start this book all over again.

Nuts, for example, are a great source of healthy fat and protein. So we think to ourselves, "This must be good for me!" A 100-calorie serving size of almonds is about 14 individual pieces. The problem is, when was the last time you counted the number of nuts you ate?

Normally we just grab a handful or, worse, eat out of the bag. We don't stop at 14 individual pieces; we stop when we're satisfied. That usually happens when we're staring at the bottom of the bag.

At that point, you've probably eaten a day's worth of fat, and everything else becomes a surplus on top of that. This is why people can't seem to lose weight even though they think they're eating "healthy" food.

If you want to lose body fat, you need to be at a caloric deficit.

But how do we know when we're finally at a deficit? Most people don't. Most people just freestyle this part. I used to be deathly afraid of carbs because I thought that if I ate too many of them, I'd get fat. At one point, I was eating half a cup of rice in total per day. I was actually severely undereating even though I thought I was eating healthy.

Again, this is the dirty work that most people ignore or simply don't know how to do.

The next question then becomes, how do we know when we're finally at a caloric deficit? Simple. It starts by figuring out our fat loss (caloric deficit) calories.

You can do it in two ways.

Option #1: Manually – Multiply Your Body Weight (in Pounds) by 9–14

Your fat loss calories will depend on your gender and your activity level [54–58]. Here's a few scenarios.

If you're a female and you have a job that requires you to sit a lot and you work out four to five times per week, then you're in the lower end of the range (9–10). If you live a fairly active lifestyle on top of regularly working out four to five times per week, then you're in the mid range (10–12).

If you're a male with an office job, then you start at the mid range (10–12). If you're active and you regularly work out, then you're in the upper range (12–14).

This number will change depending on the type of lifestyle you're currently living.

For example, if you're a fairly active individual and for some reason you get sent to Alaska for work and you're barely able to exercise, then your daily calorie intake should reflect that.

Once you have your fat loss calories, then we need to figure out your macros, short for macronutrients.

Macros are what make up the caloric content of the food we eat, and they're made up of three categories:

1. Protein

2. Carbs

3. Fat

Each macronutrient contains a certain number of calories per gram, and it's what's gonna make up your fat loss calories that we figured out earlier.

1. Protein contains 4 calories per 1 gram.

For example, 50 grams of protein equals 200 calories (50 × 4 = 200).

2. Carbs contain 4 calories per 1 gram.

For example, 50 grams of carbs equals 200 calories (50 × 4 = 200).

3. Fat contains 9 calories per 1 gram.

For example, 50 grams of fat equals 450 calories (50 × 9 = 450).

What stands out right away is that fat is the most calorie-dense macronutrient out of all three. That's important because it's something that's easy to overindulge in.

In fact, we do it *all the time*—from simple things like putting too much butter on our toast, snacking on nuts, putting too much dressing on our salad, getting a side of dipping sauce like ranch when we eat chicken wings, treating ourselves to one too many chocolate bars. The list goes on.

This isn't meant to demonize one macronutrient over the other. You need to have a healthy balance of all three to maintain optimal health and just a general sense of satisfaction whenever we eat. But you need to know how much of it you're consuming. You need to know what you're putting in your body.

Protein's Role in Fat Loss

I mentioned earlier that fat loss from intermittent fasting doesn't come from muscle. But there's one catch. You need to be in some form of resistance training. You need to work out.

Resistance training combined with eating sufficient protein prevents your muscles from withering away. Plus, protein is delicious.

How Much Protein Do You Need?

There's a lot of information out there about how much daily protein you actually need. Unless you're a professional athlete, you don't need to worry about eating a cow to satisfy your protein needs. If you're vegan and you're reading this, I'm sorry.

According to Aadam from Physiqonomics, going with 0.6 grams per pound of body weight is enough for the general population [54]. This means that if you weigh 200 pounds, 120 grams should suffice (200 grams × 0.6).

If you don't want to do the math, another way of doing it is just eating your body weight in pounds (1 gram × body weight). This means that if you weigh 125 pounds like me, then you'll want to eat 125 grams of protein every day. Lightweight, I know.

If you have *a lot* of weight to lose, then you might want to stick with the first method.

What About Carbs and Fat?

This book isn't about strict dieting, so I'm not gonna tell you that you should delete carbs from your diet or that fat is bad for you. They're both delicious.

Going on a high-carb or high-fat diet is very subjective depending on your personal preference. Just pick one that you're going to enjoy.

To borrow from Physiqonomics again, you want to set your fat intake between 0.3 and 0.6 grams per pound. For example, if you want a high-carb diet, then you want to be on the lower range of fat intake (0.3 grams per pound) and vice versa [54].

Once you figure out your fat and protein intake, then the remaining calories will be allotted to your carb intake.

Let's use my daily macros to give you a real-life example.

Carlo – body weight: 125 pounds

1. Set your fat loss calories

Fat loss calories = body weight × 9–14

I'm very active and I train six days a week, so I'm going to be on the higher end of the scale (14):

125 × 14 = 1750 calories

My calorie intake per day if I want to lose fat is 1750 calories.

2. Set your protein intake

As I mentioned earlier, to keep things simple, I'm just going to use my body weight in pounds to set my protein intake.

125 pounds = 125 grams of protein

3. Set your fat intake

Because I like to eat rice (I was born in the Philippines after all) and I also like to put butter on my toast, I'm going on the mid range for my fat intake at 0.5 grams per pound (0.3–0.6 grams per pound).

125 pounds × 0.5 grams per pound = 62.5 grams of fat or 63 grams to make things easy.

4. Set your carb intake

To calculate my total carb intake, we're going to use my protein and fat intake and figure out what they're worth in calories. Once I have those numbers, I can then figure out the number of calories I need for my carb intake and just convert that into grams.

Here's how you do it.

There are 4 calories per gram of protein, so 125 grams of protein × 4 = 500 calories from protein.

There are 9 calories per gram of fat, so 63 grams of fat × 9 = 567 calories from fat.

We now need to add those two numbers together and subtract it from my daily fat loss calories. Once we do that, we'll get my calories in carbs. Here's how:

500 calories (protein) + 567 calories (fat) = 1067 calories.

1750 calories (fat loss calories) − 1067 calories (fat + protein calories) = 683 calories.

I now have 683 calories allotted for carbs.

The last step is to convert that number into grams. We know that there are 4 calories per gram of carb, so 683 calories / 4 calories per gram of carb = 170.75 grams or 171 grams to make things easy

So my total calories and daily macros look like this:

Body weight: 125 pounds soaking wet

Daily fat loss calories: 1750 calories

125 grams of protein

63 grams of fat

171 grams of carbs

What the Heck Do I Do with Those Numbers?

I hope I didn't lose you when we did all those math calculations. But if you followed along and you figured out your own numbers using the example above, then it's time to figure out what the heck you're supposed to eat using your fat loss numbers.

Short answer?

It's up to you.

Listen, I'm not gonna sit here and tell what you can and can't eat. I'm not going to demonize one food group and hail the other as the second coming of Jesus. We all have different preferences when it comes to food.

Someone reading this book who's from Asia will have a completely different food preference over someone living in North America. Different cultures, different types of food.

What I am going to ask you to do is, before you put food in your mouth, I want you to look at the back of the packaging and look at the Nutritional Facts section—specifically, the suggested serving size. If it's not available, then look it up online. We live in a world where information is available within seconds, right at your fingertips. Use it to your advantage. You have a certain number of calories and macros that you need to fill out every day, and your food just has to fit in under that umbrella.

As a general guideline, you want to aim for a 40/30/30 split: 40% fat, 30% carbs, and 30% protein. Your fat and carb percentages are interchangeable depending on whether you want to be in a high-fat or high-carb diet. If you have a lot of fat to lose, I recommend going on a more high-fat diet in order to limit the number of carbs you consume. The less glucose in your blood from eating carbs, the faster you can start using your own body fat as a source of fuel.

But you have to be smart about how you budget your daily calorie allowance. If you use up your entire day's worth of calories on a whole pizza for lunch, then the next thing you put in your mouth will put you at a caloric surplus. If you want to stay at a caloric deficit, then you'll just have to go to sleep for dinner that day.

You can have your cake and eat it, too. But you can't have the entire cake. You have to be sensible about this. This is where moderation comes in. Just because you can doesn't mean you should.

This is where it gets tricky. Admittedly, this is why I didn't keep track of my macros for the longest time. It was just way too tedious to figure out all my numbers.

Now, if you don't want to do all that math, I'm going to introduce you to a free, powerful tool that's going to change your life. This is the "No Diet" Diet secret sauce. All you need is a smartphone and an Internet connection.

Option #2: Using MyFitnessPal

MyFitnessPal is one of the most popular health and fitness apps on the planet. It's a free online calorie calculator that tracks your macros depending on your height, weight, goals, and level of activity. Rumor has it that God didn't really rest on the seventh day; he was busy creating MyFitnessPal.

The best feature of the app is probably its Food Diary section. It's an extensive library of basically every type of food you can possibly think of. It takes the guessing game out of your diet.

You can't control what you can't measure. Now we have a tool to do just that.

How to Use MyFitnessPal:

1. Go to the app store on your phone and download the app.

2. Log in using your Facebook account. You can also create an account using your email.

3. The app is going to ask you two questions once you open it: "How much do you weigh?" and "How much would you like to weigh?" Answer as best you can. You can always change this later.

4. Now pick type of lifestyle you live: sedentary, lightly active, active, or very active. Be honest, as this will affect your daily calorie intake. Again, you can always change this later.

5. Enter you gender, height, and age.

And voila! MyFitnessPal will calculate your daily macros based on all the information you provided.

Your job then is to simply log your daily food intake. All you have to do is look up the type of food you're going to eat and its serving size using the Food Diary section. MyFitnessPal will then automatically subtract every food you log in from your daily macros and tell you how many calories you have left for the day.

Once you're happy with your weight, you can simply adjust your goal on the app to maintain that weight.

If you want a detailed, step-by-step guide on how to set up and use MyFitnessPal, you can check out my free tutorial on my YouTube channel, Newbie Fitness Academy. Don't forget to subscribe!

You see, there *is* a world where you *can* eat whatever you want. But there is a catch. There's no free pass here. In order for everything to be on the table (literally), you have to track how much of it you're putting in your body. You also have to take small breaks from eating, which we discussed earlier in this book.

Want to eat Snickers every day? Go ahead. Calamari? Chinese roast pork? Rice? Pancakes with maple syrup? Meatballs? Rice chips? You can have it all. Why do I mention those food specifically? Because those are the types of food I choose to enjoy every day. They all fit into my daily macros allowance.

If you want to see a snapshot of my food diary. Just go to:

>>> www.newbiefitnessacademy.com/dailymacros

If you don't do this, your diet is always going to be a guessing game. That's why it's so important to figure out daily calorie allowance. Better yet, let MyFitness-Pal do all the hard work for you. All you have to do is plan ahead, figure out what type of food you want to eat, figure out how much of it you want to consume, log it into your food diary, make sure you stay within your calorie allowance, and you're good to go.

You'll quickly realize that crushing a full pizza might not be such a good idea because it'll most likely take up all your calorie allowance for the day. But maybe you can squeeze a slice or two into your calorie budget so you can still enjoy yourself. Maybe a plate of spaghetti and meatballs might not be the most balanced meal after all. You'll find out quickly that restaurant portions can actually feed a small village.

This is how you can still eat whatever you want as long as it fits within your daily macros allowance.

Here's the "No Diet" Diet equation one more time:

Intermittent Fasting + Tracking Your Macros = Lean Sexy Body

You now know the benefits of intermittent fasting. You finally know how to track your macros. Do this consistently over time and you're well on your way to finally having a lean and sexy body.

You have it in you to succeed. It just involves a little bit of dirty work. But hey, you're worth it.

ACTION STEP

Download MyFitnessPal on your phone and start logging in your numbers. Have fun!

Part 4: Exercise

"The best things in life make you sweaty."
– Edgar Allan Poe

Chapter 15: You Can't Skip This Part

We're almost at the finish line.

I'm gonna give you the one and only concept you need to understand about physical health, in case you're one of those people who thinks you can just live your life and not exercise.

If you want to improve your overall health and fitness, there isn't a lot of things you can do better than to make yourself as physically strong as humanly possible.

The best way to achieve this is through strength training.

Think about the people that have made the cover of fitness magazines. A few names come to mind right away: Arnold Schwarzenegger, Michael Phelps, Tom Brady, Lebron James, Rich Froning, Serena Williams, etc.

What do all those names have in common? Other than the fact that they're icons in their respective sports, they are also in peak physical shape. They've put thousands of hours into their offseason strength and conditioning training to get where they're at today. They're ready to go to war once the clock starts.

If you go back to our hunter-gatherer days, the people that were able to hunt and provide were the ones that survived and prospered. That ones that couldn't? They probably got eaten alive by a lion or a bear. In order to be effective hunters, they needed to be fast and they definitely needed to be strong. Have you ever tried hauling a dead deer? Yeah, me neither. But they look heavy as hell.

Because here's the thing—I mentioned in the last chapter that there's a catch in order for you not to lose muscle when you fast. The "No Diet" Diet hinges on you being in some form of resistance training.

You need to work out. Yes, I know you're busy. This is such a sticking point for a lot of people, especially those who have never worked out before or had bad experiences with it.

It can be very intimidating. Trust me, I know how it feels. I've been there before. When I first started, I had what some people call "spaghetti arms." I couldn't do a single pull-up. I could barely move a 45-pound barbell over my head. I couldn't lift anything respectable if my life depended on it. I also ate a lot of spaghetti. Maybe that had something to do with it.

If it makes you feel better, just remember that every expert was once a beginner. Yes, even Arnold

Schwarzenegger. Or maybe he was already born with abs. Who knows?

One of the biggest benefits of working out, other than looking good shirtless, is that it builds your overall functional strength. If you can build your overall functional strength, it's going to be a lot easier to be a more functional human being. You can climb a tree and rescue a kitten, you can pull yourself out of a burning building, or you can play catch with your kid, if you have one, without throwing out your back. This goes all the way down to simple tasks like being able to carry your groceries.

At the end of the day, I think that's what fitness is all about—being a more functional human being.

This Might Be the Worst Way to Get Fit

Raise your hand if you've spent any sort of time on a treadmill or an elliptical machine or if you've ever gone to a spin class.

Did you get a good sweat? Maybe. Maybe not.

As with most diets, most of the information about working out is outdated, misleading, or just plain wrong and silly.

For example, long-duration cardio like running, spending an ungodly amount of time on the elliptical machine, the Stairmaster, or those ridiculously expensive spinning classes are not very good for you, despite their popularity.

They're trendy, but they don't help you lose weight very effectively and have a very poor ratio of results to time spent, particularly if that's all you're doing for exercise.

Yet a lot of people are still under the belief that spending a stupid amount of time doing cardio will somehow get them a raging six pack.

Nothing, and I mean *nothing,* could be further from the truth.

Running, for example, is the most popular exercise on earth after walking. The problem is, it's unbelievably inefficient when it comes to burning fat and building muscle. What's worse is that up to 79% of runners get injured at least once a year [55]. That's almost eight out of every 10 people hobbling around from what is considered a "safe" exercise.

It's one of the easiest things to do when you're just starting out. I'll give it that. It's convenient. How easy is it to just lace up your runners and hop on the treadmill and hit the start button? It takes no effort and almost zero technique.

But it's lazy and extremely inefficient.

How to Work Out Smarter

The best exercises are the ones that improve your life outside of the gym—whether that means moving furniture around your house and jumping across an obstacle to more drastic situations like pulling your own body weight over a fence so you can save yourself from a burning building and being able to outrun a bear.

Okay, that last one was a lie. You can't outrun a bear. I don't care if your name is Usain Bolt. Black and grizzly bears can outrun any human on any terrain. Good luck with that.

Those exercises are what I like to call functional, and for the most part, they require free weights.

Free weights allow your body to move throughout all three planes of motion (lateral, frontal, axial) because they aren't fixed to a certain path [56]. Think about a kettlebell swing or an Olympic weightlifting movement like the snatch. The weights and your body move freely throughout the movement.

Your larger muscles, stabilizer muscles, and core all have to work together to control your movements. This means that with every rep you're strengthening way more than one muscle. The more muscle you work during a given exercise, the more calories you're going to burn with every rep.

When you do a shoulder press, your shoulders, core, and posterior chain all have to work together to stabilize the barbell over your head. Another example is a classic compound movement, such as the deadlift. It seamlessly carries over to daily activities like lifting grocery or shopping bags—the definition of functional fitness.

The KISS Principle

Your body includes 206 bones and as many as 840 skeletal muscles. To build your overall functional strength as quickly and efficiently as possible, you want to involve as many of these skeletal muscles as you possibly can. The problem is, most people can only identify a handful of these muscles: abs, more abs, pecs, and biceps.

Compound movements like pull-ups, shoulder presses, squats, and deadlifts use dozens of muscles to stabilize and move multiple joints. And for the most part, they use free weights. Movements that fall into this category closely resemble the actions of daily life. If you are a beginner and want the most time-efficient workouts, you should use your time focusing on basic compound movements.

Ever heard of the KISS principle? It's a design princi-ple by the U.S. Navy in the 1960s. It's an acronym for "keep it simple, stupid." It speaks for itself. You want to make your workouts as simple as possible.

No, you don't need to step on a Bosu ball with a barbell on your back when you do your squats. That's just an injury waiting to happen. The weights you're able to lift will pale in comparison if you just squat from the rack like a normal, non-douchy human being.

You also need to stop thinking about separate body parts. You can't just spot treat yourself. You can't just say, "I'm gonna do 100 sit-ups a day to get a six pack." You may or may not get there—I'm not quite sure. But that is an unbelievably inefficient way of doing it.

Combine this with intermittent fasting and tracking your macros and you're well on your way to burning fat, building muscle, and building a body you're proud of. There, I just gave you the secret to life.

You Don't Need Machines; You Are the Machine

It seems like every commercial gym is loaded with treadmills, ellipticals, Stairmasters, and exercise ma-chines aimed to hit every individual muscle you have.

A lot of people also find the weirdest and funniest ways to use these aforementioned machines, mostly because they don't know how. That's how those funny gym videos you find all over the Internet are born.

For most people starting out, the gym can be a very intimidating place. The simple act of showing up is half the battle. I mentioned at the beginning of this book that my first gym experience wasn't really the most pleasant one. My brother basically had to drag me, kicking and screaming, to the local YMCA because I didn't want to go. I was terrified I was going to make a fool of myself in front of everyone there (I did).

That's why people tend to gravitate toward the cardio area, then make their way over to the exercise machines. Why? Because it's the easiest thing to get started with. At least they look like the "safest" way to lift weights. You just look at the instructions and then instant fitness happens! Right??

Unfortunately, nothing could be further from the truth.

When you use a machine, your body is forced to move on a single, unilateral direction. The problem is, your body doesn't move that way. Machines also lure you into a false sense of security because they do all the stabilization work for you.

Let's use the Smith machine, for example. People think it's a "safe" machine to use for squats, but that statement couldn't be more wrong.

The machine only travels along a fixed path, not allowing you to use any natural movement or core engagement when you squat. Your knees wind up in front of you as you descend to your bottom squat position, which decreases the involvement of your hamstrings. This creates a shearing force at the joint, which is bad news for your patella tendon. In layman's terms, it's bad for your knees.

You also see a lot of people squat stupid amounts of weight using this machine yet struggle to squat a light barbell from the rack.

Your specialty when you're at the gym is to not specialize in anything. You want to be a well-rounded, fully functional human being, and your training should reflect that—from simple tasks like picking up groceries, helping a friend move, playing sports on the weekend, all the way to being able to pull somebody out of a burning building. You want to make sure that you have access to all the tools in your physical toolbox and can perform any of those tasks at the snap of a finger.

Unless you're an elite bodybuilder or you're rehabbing an injury, you do not need to concern yourself with machines. Stick with free weights and compound movements where you'll get the best return on your time investment.

Here's the summary of this chapter so far in one paragraph in case you got lazy and you've just been mindlessly flipping through this book:

You need to lift weights. Don't use machines. You are the machine. No, I don't expect you to break the deadlift world record. If you're a girl reading this and you think that you're going to look like an ancient Amazon warrior from lifting weights, then I need you to pump the brakes for a second. Here are two perfectly valid reasons why you won't:

1. It'll takes months, if not years of strict dieting and sticking to a regimented workout plan for you to develop that type of physique.
2. What's wrong with having muscles? Strong is the new sexy.

This Is the Type of Workout You Should Do

Time is one of our most precious resources. You can always make more money but you can't make more time.

One of the most common excuses that people have for why they don't work out is that they don't have time. I get it. You're busy. The last thing that you want to do after a long day at work is go to a crowded gym.

But what if I told you that you don't need to spend countless hours at the gym to get results?

Instead of working out longer and doing a million isolation movements and using every single exercise machine, I want you to work out smarter by doing intervals of high-intensity compound movements alternating with short rests done repeatedly.

This type of workout is called HIIT, short for high-intensity interval training. A lot of evidence shows that HIIT, and other forms of it, is amazingly effective at getting you results in as little time as possible [57].

If you have time to read a book or watch TV while you're working out, then you're doing it wrong.

Fitness programs like CrossFit, boot camps, and even Barre classes are very effective at implementing HIIT workouts. Joining a group fitness class is also a great way to socialize and meet like-minded people.

If you're not ready to sign up for a gym membership just yet or your local gym doesn't offer any group fitness classes, try out this short but highly effective bodyweight workout. All you need is a small space, a little motivation, and a good attitude! Did I mention it's only eight minutes long?

Beginner Bodyweight Tabata Workout (Tabata: 20 seconds on; 10 seconds off)

4 rounds of:

Sit-ups

Push-ups

Burpees

Squats

Want a free demo of the workout? Just go to:

>>> www.newbiefitnessacademy.com/freedemo

Note: The movements we used for this workout are part of the Ultimate Bodyweight Movement Cheatsheet. The cheatsheet reveals the only eight bodyweight movements that you'll need in order to find a fitter, leaner, and more awesome version of you.

It doesn't have to be complicated for it to be effective. To download your free copy, just go to:

>>> www.newbiefitnessacademy.com/cheatsheet

The key is to push through the high-intensity intervals (for 20 seconds) and lower your heart rate during the 10-second rest.

The biggest thing you have to remember is that the intensity is always relative to the person doing it, meaning if you have to do push-ups off your knees or on your desk, then that's your starting point, and you just progress from there.

If you want more free workouts, just head over to my YouTube Channel, Newbie Fitness Academy. That's where I post short but highly effective workouts once a week. It doesn't matter if you're just starting out or if you're a seasoned pro. Make sure you subscribe so you can stay up to date with the weekly workouts. All you have to do is show up and just follow along.

How Often Should You Work Out?

If you're new to this whole fitness thing, try to rest for 48 hours in between workouts to give your body enough time to recover. You're new. It's probably gonna feel like you just got hit by a bus the next day after doing your first workout.

Once your body adapts to your new workout program, you can go on a two-days-on and one-day-off cycle. If you have extra time, you can even take it a step further and go three days on and one day off.

The key to all this is to find a time and schedule that works for you. The best workout plan is the one that's sustainable and fits in your life seamlessly.

Chapter 16: Action Always Beats Intention

"For what it's worth: It's never too late to be whoever you want to be. I hope you live a life you're proud of. If you find that you're not, I hope you have the courage to start all over again." – Eric Roth

I don't really know how to properly end this book, so I guess we can just start with that quote.

I've also been talking about dieting and fitness this entire time, but we haven't really defined what it actually means. So I guess we can talk about that next.

The dictionary defines the word fitness as the condition of being physically fit and healthy.

Physically fit but, most importantly, healthy. I think everybody can get behind that. Having a six pack is great, but at the end of the day, you want to do this to improve your quality of life, and being healthy is key when it comes to that.

Here's the "No Diet" Diet equation one last time:

Intermittent Fasting + Tracking Your Macros = Lean Sexy Body

Once we add sleep and exercise to that equation, then it becomes the "No Diet" lifestyle to a physically fit and healthy body:

Sleep (7–9 hours) + Intermittent Fasting (16-hour fast) + Tracking Your Macros (MyFitnessPal) + Exercise (HIIT Workouts) = Lean Sexy Body

That's it. If you follow that equation, then you can turn this entire thing into a healthy lifestyle for the rest of your life. Imagine finally having your dream body without giving up your favorite food.

Remember the KISS principle? Always keep things simple. Don't overcomplicate it. Focus on taking things one day at a time and know that it's gonna take some time. Focus on making one good decision at a time. Small daily good decisions done repeatedly add up to staggering results over time.

Accept that you're bound to stumble once or twice. Fall in love with the process and know that there's gonna be some rainy days. Just pick yourself back up, pull up your socks, and keep chipping away.

Nothing worth having ever comes easy. You might even think you can't do this. Just remember that every reason why you think you can't is the reason why you have to.

"I have too much weight to lose. I don't know if I can do this."

That's exactly why you need to take action. Do you want to miss out on life because you can't get yourself out of bed? Do you want to miss out on your daughter's wedding because you have diabetes?

"I have no time."

That's exactly it. You're almost out of time. You need to do this now.

"I have a kid."

That should be your biggest motivator. You want to be a good role model for your kid that you can do this, that you can achieve something that you've never had before.

Here's my secret to all of this, and this might be the secret to a happy life as well.

You have to like what you're doing. You have to enjoy it. If not, you're not gonna last. You're gonna find every excuse to go back to your old habits.

You need to know your *why*. You have to take care of your sleep. You have to like the food you eat. You need to take small breaks from eating and track what you're putting in your body. You have to like whatever workout you're doing.

Add up all those things and fitness happens.

The Next Step

You now have everything you need to get the body you've always wanted while still eating whatever you want.

It really is that simple. Weight loss is not this complicated thing that "experts" make it out to be.

The next step is up to you. It's all about taking action now. You have it in you to succeed.

Although you have everything you need to be successful, some of you might have some additional questions and need extra help.

If that's the case, I strongly recommend you check out my online fitness program. It's where I hold your hand step by freaking step on how to implement everything I talked about in this book.

If you're serious about getting results and want to make sure you give yourself the best chance to succeed, then this program is the best vehicle for you to get there.

Think of it as driving a Tesla through your fat loss journey versus taking a tuk-tuk. You want to be in the Tesla for this.

If you want to know more about the program, go to:

>>> www.newbiefitnessacademy.com/the-next-step

Also, I'd love to hear your thoughts! If you followed the "No Diet" Diet and it changed your life completely, I'd love to hear about it! Hearing people's success stories is what motivates me to do what I do every day.

Just send me an email at <u>info@newbiefitnessacademy.com</u>.

Here's to your new healthy and sexy body.

Carlo Macapinlac

Help Me Help, Other People

Congratulations!

You've reached the last page of this book.

If you somehow skipped through the entire thing and managed to randomly land on this page, that's okay, too.

Before you go and implement everything you've learned in this book, I have one small favor to ask.

Reviews are the best way for independent authors like me to get noticed, sell more books, and spread their message to other people.

If you even got one thing or one idea from this book, that will make your life 1% better. Then I'll sleep better at night knowing I've done my job as an author.

Would you take a minute to write a review about this book on Amazon? Just type "The 'No Diet' Diet" in the search box, scroll down on the page, and hit "Write a customer review." It would mean the world to me.

You're awesome. Thank you.

The "No Diet" Diet References

1. https://www.telegraph.co.uk/women/womens-life/11915375/How-long-those-spontaneous-selfies-really-take.html

2. onlinelibrary.wiley.com/doi/10.1038/oby.2007.118/full

3. https://www.cdc.gov/media/releases/2016/p0215-enough-sleep.html

4. https://en.wikipedia.org/wiki/Obesity_in_the_United_States

5. www.ncbi.nlm.nih.gov/pmc/articles/PMC535701/

6. www.ncbi.nlm.nih.gov/pmc/articles/PMC2398753/

7. https://www.ncbi.nlm.nih.gov/pmc/articles/PMC3842900/

8. https://www.psychologytoday.com/blog/sleep-newzzz/201303/less-sleep-means-more-calories

9. https://authoritynutrition.com/how-many-calories-per-day/

10. www.ncbi.nlm.nih.gov/pmc/articles/PMC535701/

11. www.ncbi.nlm.nih.gov/pmc/articles/PMC3619301/

12. www.ncbi.nlm.nih.gov/pubmed/21300732

13. www.ncbi.nlm.nih.gov/pubmed/10543671

14. https://www.sciencedaily.com/releases/2015/01/150105081757.htm

15. https://justgetflux.com/

16. http://selfcontrolapp.com/

17. nutritiondata.self.com/facts/breakfast-cereals/1655/2

18. www.telegraph.co.uk/news/health/news/10668189/Low-fat-foods-stuffed-with-harmful-levels-of-sugar.html

19. www.ncbi.nlm.nih.gov/pubmed/17921363

20. https://www.fatsecret.com/calories-nutrition/usda/orange-juice?portionid=43802&portionamount=12.000

21. www.myfitnesspal.com/food/calories/m-ms-plain-1-bag-corrected-per-website-1-30-14-547302431

22. onlinelibrary.wiley.com/doi/10.1002/oby.21538/abstract

23. dictionary.com

24. https://en.wikipedia.org/wiki/Basal_metabolic_rate

25. https://fitfolk.com/average-basal-energy-expenditure-bee-basal-metabolic-rate-bmr/

26. www.businessinsider.com/this-one-statistic-shows-how-much-mcdonalds-tries-to-entrench-itself-in-everybodys-minds-2012-3

27. www.ncbi.nlm.nih.gov/pubmed/19566598

28. www.ncbi.nlm.nih.gov/pubmed/8172872

29. www.ncbi.nlm.nih.gov/pubmed/21051570

30. www.leangains.com/2009/12/fasted-training-boosts-muscle-growth.html

31. well.blogs.nytimes.com/2010/12/15/phys-ed-the-benefits-of-exercising-before-breakfast/

32. www.leangains.com/2010/09/fasted-training-insulin-sensitivity.html

33. www.ncbi.nlm.nih.gov/pmc/articles/PMC329619/?page=1

34. www.ncbi.nlm.nih.gov/pubmed/9155494

35. https://www.cdc.gov/media/releases/2017/p0718-diabetes-report.html

36. www.sciencedirect.com/science/article/pii/S193152441400200X

37. www.ncbi.nlm.nih.gov/pubmed/15640462

38. www.ncbi.nlm.nih.gov/pubmed/11319710

39. https://www.endocrine.org/news-room/press-release-archives/2010/testosteronedecreasesafteringestionofsugar

40. www.ncbi.nlm.nih.gov/pubmed/?term=Pituitary-testicular+axis+in+obese+men+during+short-term+fasting.

41. https://www.quora.com/Why-is-the-testos-terone-level-high-early-in-the-morning

42. www.ncbi.nlm.nih.gov/pmc/arti-cles/PMC329619/?page=6

43. www.ncbi.nlm.nih.gov/pmc/arti-cles/PMC2990190/

44. https://aax-us-east.amazon-adsys-tem.com/x/c/Qq6LWegKHUFAO2lYGknU-uMsAAAFhuP4JAQEAAAF-KAaQs3YY/http://www.amazon.com/Mis-guided-Medicine-ill-advised-medical-recom-mendations/dp/1500675385/ref=as_at?crea-tiveASIN=1500675385&linkCode=w50&tag=grtist-20&imprTo-ken=YlLU2xBsqEOsLQH.AwN-hhw&slotNum=0

45. https://www.dietdoctor.com/renew-body-fast-ing-autophagy

46. jn.nutrition.org/content/31/3/363.full.pdf

47. www.karger.com/Article/Abstract/212538

48. ajcn.nutrition.org/content/86/1/7.full

49. www.ncbi.nlm.nih.gov/pubmed/18184721

50. www.bornfitness.com/how-to-fight-aging

51. http://www.eatstopeat.com/

52. https://leangains.com/

53. https://leangains.com/questions-answers/

54. http://physiqonomics.com/the-best-fat-loss-ar-ticle-child-friendly-version/

55. bjsm.bmj.com/content/bjsports/41/8/469.full.pdf

56. athletics.wikia.com/wiki/Planes_of_Motion

57. https://www.acefitness.org/education-and-resources/lifestyle/blog/5073/8-reasons-hiit-workouts-are-so-effective

58. https://bodyrecomposition.com/

Made in the USA
San Bernardino, CA
09 May 2018